Understanding, Assessing & Treating Dentomandibular Sensorimotor Dysfunction

Understanding, Assessing & Treating Dentomandibular Sensorimotor Dysfunction

With contributions by:
Allison M. DiMatteo, BA, MPS
Mark W. Montgomery, DMD

With forward by:
Roger P. Levin, DDS

*Understanding, Assessing & Treating
Dentomandibular Sensorimotor Dysfunction*

Managing & Contributing Editor: Allison DiMatteo, BA, MPS

Book Design: Katelyn Bartman
　　　　　　Crème della Crème Copywriting & Communication

Cover Design: Deanna Murphy
　　　　　　　Dental Resource Systems, Inc.

Cover Image Credits: Purchased from INMAGINE®

Other Image Credits: See page 141

Copyright © 2012 by Dental Resource Systems, Inc.
All rights reserved. No part of this publication may be reproduced or transmitted in any form or by any means, electronic or mechanical, including photocopying, recording, or any information storage and retrieval system, without permission in writing from Dental Resource Systems, Inc. Permissions may be sought directly from Dental Resource Systems, Inc.: 1700 E. Las Olas Blvd., Suite 300, Fort Lauderdale, FL, 33301; Phone: 855-770-4002.

Notice: *Knowledge and best practice in dentistry are constantly changing. As new research and experience broaden the profession's knowledge, changes in practice, treatment, and therapy become necessary or appropriate. Readers are advised to check the most current information provided on procedures discussed or the products to be used or administered to verify the recommended method and usage and any contraindications. It is the responsibility of the practitioner, relying on their own experience and knowledge of the patient, to make diagnoses and assessments, and to determine the best treatment for each individual patient, and to take all appropriate safety precautions. To the fullest extent of the law, neither Dental Resource Systems, Inc., nor the Authors, Editors, or Reviewers, assumes any liability for any injury and/or damage to persons or property arising out of or related to any use of the material contained in this book.--- Dental Resource Systems, Inc.*

CONTRIBUTORS

Allison M. DiMatteo, BA, MPS

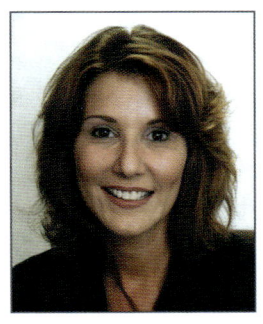

Allison DiMatteo is the founder and owner of Crème della Crème Copywriting & Communication, a consulting firm in upstate New York specializing in professional journalism, publication editing and management, graphic design and identity, and marketing, public relations, and customer communication. Clients include dental product and equipment manufacturers, laboratories, dentists, professional and civic organizations, and businesses in the publishing and consumer industries.

A regular contributor to **Inside Dentistry** magazine, she also is the manuscript development liaison for the **Journal of Cosmetic Dentistry**, the official publication of the American Academy of Cosmetic Dentistry (AACD). Ms. DiMatteo also served for three years as the editor of **Consumer Guide to Dentistry**, an online publication for consumers seeking quality dental information. Additionally, she has lectured about writing case presentations for peer-review publication for such venues as the AACD Annual Scientific Session, as well as on other communication topics for various education and training programs.

Ms. DiMatteo is a graduate of Nazareth College of Rochester with a BA in English and Cornell University with an MPS in Communication. A member of the Board of Directors for the Cayuga County Chamber of Commerce, she writes and consults on strategies for collateral materials, marketing programs, advertisements, corporate scripts, and other content for numerous businesses.

CONTRIBUTORS

Mark W. Montgomery, DMD

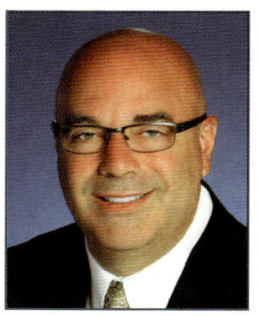

Dr. Mark W. Montgomery has been committed to excellent patient care since graduating from Oregon Health Sciences University in 1980. His experience in all aspects of dental care has been enhanced by extensive work in continuing dental education. This background has built a strong commitment to comprehensive health grounded in beautiful smiles, excellent chewing function, and a health/biological focus.

Dr. Montgomery has lectured and taught extensively regarding dentomandibular sensorimotor function and dysfunction. He has developed integrated systems to manage pain, headaches, temporomandibular joint disorders, and force managed occlusion. He has taught thousands of dentists to use well-defined systems to enhance their clinical excellence.

He is well-known for his mastery of skills in Invisalign orthodontics, smile enhancements and veneers, reconstruction and restoration of worn and damaged teeth, and in controlling tooth grinding, dentomandibular sensorimotor dysfunction, and head/face pain.

Dr. Montgomery currently teaches live patient hands-on curricula for post-graduate clinical studies in the areas of pain, headaches, sensorimotor dysfunction, occlusion, and full-mouth reconstruction. He also is Chief Dental Officer at Dental Resource Systems, and has been an educator with Pride Institute, PAC~live, the Hornbrook Group, and Aesthetic Masters in the area of Clinical Management. Dr. Montgomery was formerly on the faculty of AlignTech Institute, training dentists in the Invisalign system.

EDITORIAL BOARD

Richard Amy

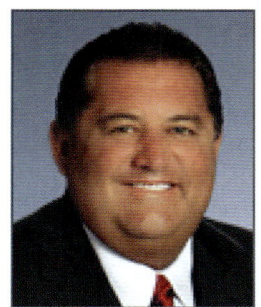

Dr. Richard Amy is an instructor, educator, researcher, author, inventor, and innovator in the health care arena. His pioneering efforts have resulted in treatment-specific approaches that focus on functional neurological restoration.

Having worked with clinical trial design and reporting metrics, his prior efforts resulted in the first Food and Drug Administration (FDA) clearance for the therapeutic uses of low level lasers. Since that time, he has catapulted his neurological healing applications, using lasers and other modalities, to a number of specific areas of pioneering interest.

His background includes broad experience in neurology, orthopedics, general medicine, dentistry, nutrition, rehabilitation, and molecular sciences. This gives him a well-rounded foundation for the treatment and correction of many maladies.

Dr. Amy has been an instructor for functional neurology correction across many health care disciplines. He incorporates the accepted standard for care and objective diagnostic metrics to prove his safe and non-invasive methods. During the last two decades, he has not only instructed professionally, but has volunteered his time at clinics and hospitals across the globe.

Over the last several years, he has focused much of his research efforts on dentistry and provided instruction for dental practitioners, including specialists and surgeons, on a number of neurologically related problems affecting the head, neck, and mouth. Early detection of the signs and symptoms can allow for relatively simple correction. His work may well prove to be one of the most significant advancements in dentistry for the 21st century.

EDITORIAL BOARD

Martin Jablow, DMD

Dr. Martin Jablow presents and publishes worldwide on many topics, including state-of-the-art dental technology and dental materials. A clinician, speaker, and author, he is president of Dental Technology Solutions, a lecture and consulting company.

Dr. Jablow graduated from Rutgers University and, in 1986, received his dental degree from University of Medicine and Dentistry of New Jersey. He practices general dentistry in a group setting in Woodbridge, NJ.

An active member of the American Dental Association, New Jersey Dental Association, and Middlesex County Dental Association, Dr. Jablow achieved Fellowships in the Academy of General Dentistry and International Academy of Dental Facial Esthetics. For more than 20 years, he has been a member of his local peer review and was an attending dentist at the John F. Kennedy Medical Center in Edison, NJ, where he worked with patients and trained residents.

Dr. Jablow's recurring columns can be found on DrBicuspid.com and Dental-LearningHub.com's *Apex Magazine*. He serves on the Dentalcompare CE Advisory Board, as well as the Eco-Dentistry Association Advisory Board. As the Internet has grown, so has Dr. Jablow's online presence with his dental blog, webinars, and as host of TakeFiveWithMarty.com.

EDITORIAL BOARD

Roger P. Levin, DDS

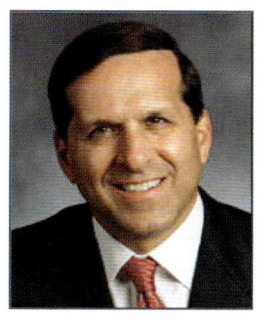

Dr. Roger P. Levin is a third-generation general dentist and the Chairman and CEO of Levin Group, Inc., the largest dental practice consulting firm in the world. Levin Group was founded in 1985 when Dr. Levin recognized a vital missing link that was preventing his fellow dentists and specialists from increasing practice production. As a leading authority on dental practice management and marketing, he has developed the scientific systems-based consulting method that increases practice production and profitability while lowering stress.

He has authored more than 60 books and over 3,000 articles. Dr. Levin sits on the editorial boards of five prominent dental publications, serves as the practice management editor of **Compendium,** and is the managing editor of **Dental Business Review**. He is also a regular contributor to the **Journal of the American Dental Association**.

Dr. Levin has been named one of the "Leaders in Dental Consulting" by **Dentistry Today** magazine for the past 10 years. He is a past recipient of the Ernst & Young Entrepreneur of the Year award, has served on the Board of Advisors of the University of Pennsylvania, School of Dental Medicine, served as adjunct faculty for several dental schools, and is a former Chairman of the National Museum of Dentistry.

Dr. Levin presents more than 100 seminars worldwide each year and is a keynote speaker for major dental conferences. He has been interviewed by the **Wall Street Journal**, **New York Times**, and **Time Magazine**.

EDITORIAL BOARD

Ronald Ritsco, DMD, MS

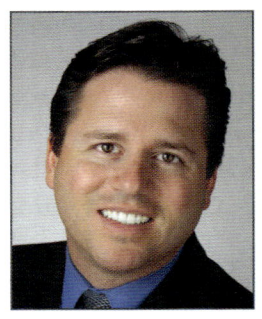

Dr. Ronald Ritsco is a prosthodontist, author, researcher, and international instructor in implants, aesthetic smile design, full-mouth rehabilitation, and temporomandibular joint disorders. He maintains a successful private practice, Ritsco Prosthodontics Advanced Dentistry, devoted to general family and specialized care. He is also the Director of the Aesthetic Masters Hands-On Courses for dentists at the University of Nevada, Las Vegas (UNLV), Dental School.

Dr. Ritsco graduated from the University of Texas Health Science Center (UTHSC) in San Antonio specializing in prosthodontics. He simultaneously earned his MS degree in prosthodontics from the School of Biomedical Graduate Sciences. An active member of the American Academy of Cosmetic Dentistry, American College of Prosthodontics, and the American Academy of Maxillofacial Prosthetics, he has received multiple honors, including the American College of Oral Medicine Award and the President's Award from the Canadian Dental Association.

Dr. Ritsco is committed to researching clinical applications of ceramics, complete dentures, and implant prosthetics, and devotes much of his time to continuing education. A former Clinical Instructor of Prosthodontics, Occlusion, and Implants in the Department of Restorative Dentistry at UTHSC at San Antonio and the University of Saskatchewan College of Dentistry, he is currently an Associate Professor at multiple accredited dental schools.

Dr. Ritsco has written numerous scientific journal articles and textbook chapters.

EDITORIAL BOARD

John Schwartz, DDS

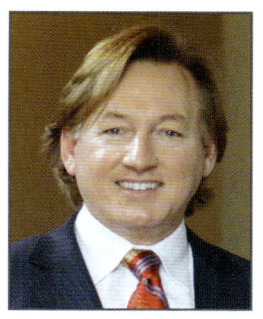

Dr. John Schwartz is a master ceramist, innovator, author, researcher, and instructor in the field of oral esthetics and dental ceramics. The inventor of the vertical shoulder preparation for porcelain laminate veneers, a technique accepted around the world as the definitive esthetic preparation technique for porcelain laminate veneers, he also is the creator/designer of the bleached dentition in ceramic. Along with others, Dr. Schwartz is a creator of the layering technique for milled and pressed laminates that is now the gold standard for porcelain veneers.

Dr. Schwartz conducts research in the strengths of ceramic crowns. The results of his work led to a fabrication technique of lithium disilicate substructures that can increase the strength of lithium disilicate supported crowns by as much as 34 percent.

In addition to maintaining his dental practice devoted to esthetics, Dr. Schwartz is the director of the Integra Institute Center for Advanced Dental Learning and an Assistant Clinical Professor at the Louisiana State University School of Dentistry, Department of Prosthodontics. He consistently ranks in the 95th percentile for excellence for his lectures and courses at dental association and dental laboratory association meetings when surveyed by attendees.

Dr. Schwartz has authored numerous articles featured in such dental publications as *Quintessence of Dental Technology*, *Inside Dentistry*, *Dentistry Today*, *Dental Products Report*, and *Practical Periodontics & Aesthetic Dentistry*. He also was featured in National Dental Network's DVD series, "Excellence in Cosmetic Dentistry", and has conducted educational videos for Integra Institute and DentalXP.

TABLE OF CONTENTS

Preface 19

Forward 23

1 *Diagnostics, Discovery and Dentistry's Expanding Capabilities* 29

- Advancements in Understanding the Greater Dentomandibular Complex 31
- Opportunities Presented by Need and Knowledge 37
- The Time Is Now 41
- References 43
- Chapter 1 Self-Assessment Quiz... 51

2 *Dentomandibular Sensorimotor Dysfunction and Its Role in Chronic Pain* 55

- Muscular and Joint Considerations 64
- Neurophysiological Considerations 66
- Implications for Dentomandibular and Headache Pain Treatments ... 69
- Embracing New Opportunities for Assessment and Therapy .. 71
- References 73
- Chapter 2 Self-Assessment Quiz... 78

3 The TruDenta System for Assessing and Treating Dentomandibular Sensorimotor Dysfunction 83

- The Scientifically Proven Components 85
- Examinations and Histories 86
- The Digital Assessment Modalities 89
  - Force Measurement 90
  - Range of Motion Assessment 92
- The Rehabilitation Modalities 94
  - Therapeutic Ultrasound 95
  - Transcutaneous Electrical Stimulation 95
  - Low Level Laser/Light Therapy 95
  - Manual Muscle/Trigger Point Therapy 97

References 98

Chapter 3 Self-Assessment Quiz 106

4 Life Changing Dentistry: Implications for the TruDenta Pathway to Care 111

- The TruDenta Rehabilitation Process 113
- Realizing Life Changing Results 117

References 120

Chapter 4 Self-Assessment Quiz 123

5 Shifting the Paradigm to Enhance Oral Health and Headache Care Effectiveness ... *127*

    References ... 132

    Chapter 5 Self-Assessment Quiz ... 133

Self-Assessment Quiz Answers ... 137

List of Tables ... 139

Image Credits ... 141

Index ... 143

Preface

Mark W. Montgomery, DMD

Richard Amy

Headaches, migraines, chronic daily headaches, tension-type headaches, myofascial pain, facial pain, temporomandibular joint disorders (TMJ/D), TMJ derangements, degenerative joint disease, malocclusion, abnormal tooth wear patterns, abfractions, parafunction, clenching, grinding, bruxism…

For many years now, dentists have been observing, studying, and treating a number of these disorders that seemed to have common etiologies and patho-physiologies rooted in the sensorimotor processing of the trigeminal nerve and related cranial nerves. Now, the latest research in the neuroscience of the trigeminal nucleus bears out the observations, suspicions, and treatment efforts of these dentists, so much so that we can now begin to group many of these disorders into a category that we call dentomandibular sensorimotor dysfunction.

These dysfunctions are the result of the direct interplay of the neuronal and non-neuronal activity of the trigeminal nucleus with the musculature of the head and neck. This is the oral therapeutic care we dentists live everyday when managing the stomatognathic function of our patients.

Sensorimotor and somatosensory functions are inextricably linked to protective reflexes, hormonal responses, and the neurology that is at the heart of immunology and inflammation. Trauma, stress, chronic inflammation, medication overuse, and dysfunction are combining at an alarming rate and causing severe lifestyle disease in our patients. Under these conditions, pain becomes the disease we know as chronic pain (i.e., centrally mediated pain, central sensitization). Chronic pain becomes a neurochemical negative feedback loop that perpetuates dysfunction and neuro-inflammation. This then leads to neurotransmitter disorders that can manifest as headache, migraine, depression, anxiety, insomnia, and other lifestyle coping mechanisms that damage and destroy our patients' lives (and their teeth).

And all of this is happening right under our noses.

- Pain processed in the trigeminal nucleus.

- Pain travelling the trigeminal thalamic tract.

- Affecting and affected by the glial cell modulation in the trigeminal ganglion and the trigeminal nucleus.

- With cross-connected communication in the facial, glossopharyngeal, vagus, and accessory cranial nerves.

- Correlated with proprioceptive feedback and sensorimotor function.

- Affected by abnormal function and trigger point pain and referred pain.

- And, maybe most importantly, able to be influenced by re-establishing normal function of the dentomandibular sensorimotor system.

    o Including normal ranges of motion of the mandible and the upper neck.

    o Including normal envelope of function and force balance of the dentition.

Our previous systems for treating headaches and pain have included re-establishing mandibular position and careful interdigitation of the dentition. We have used a variety of modalities, such as orthotics, orthodontics, myofascial release, physical therapy, restorative dentistry, etc. These have all enjoyed a modicum of success and have been utilized in a somewhat symptom-driven, trial and error approach by many dentists. Until now, though, the comprehensive rehabilitation therapy approach has not been used effectively to get at the heart of the dysfunction and sensorimotor influence.

As you'll see in this volume, this comprehensive, calibrated, combination approach to assessing and rehabilitating the dentomandibular sensorimotor function is the most thorough, effective, and conservative system to date. It can be used when nothing else has worked. It can be used at the time of initial injury. It can be used as a first line of therapy to avoid costly and extensive invasive procedures, where possible. And it can be used to get at the heart of pain and headaches. Having a system like this brings new hope for the patients suffering from the many various maladies associated with these pervasive problems. This system is truly the missing link in dental medicine today.

We wish great success in health and health care for you and your patients.

Mark W. Montgomery, DMD

Richard Amy

Forward

By Roger P. Levin, DDS

Chairman and Chief Executive Officer

Levin Group, Inc.

It's an exciting time to be in dentistry and the oral healthcare profession. The future holds tremendous promise with the advent of technologies that enhance the quality of care provided to patients. As digital technologies gain wider acceptance, new equipment is increasingly becoming commonplace in practice. This equipment includes CAD/CAM, digital radiographs, oral cancer screening devices, digital impression taking, lasers, and caries detection systems. Innovative technologies entering the market that have the potential to enable dental professionals to offer wonderful new treatments are as equally important.

However, a challenge facing many of today's practicing dentists is balancing subjective judgments with objective decision-making. Contributing to this dilemma has been a lack of complete and properly applied assessment tools, all of which can be systematically incorporated into the practice to formulate treatment plans to an accurate and unbiased standard of care.

As an advocate of technology in the dental practice, I have long advised dentists to evaluate their technology options to ensure that they can satisfy any combination of four criteria in order to be worthwhile. First, technologies should improve the speed with which the dental team can comprehensively address a patient's concerns or deliver treatment. Secondly, technology should improve the quality of that treatment. Third, it should increase the dental team's effectiveness. Finally, technology should provide a return on investment. Although some technologies might be considered a significant investment, they can represent an excellent return when incorporated into everyday use.

When a technology satisfies one or more of these criteria, a dental practice can then confidently proceed to developing a systematic plan. This plan is meant to integrate the technology into the practice. Additionally, technologies that have a proven track record for success and clinical application, based on research and literature, lend support to their integration in practice.

Of paramount importance to achieving a successful technology integration is ensuring that effective systems are in place to increase overall practice production, especially within the current patient base. Highly efficient systems enable dentists and their teams to maximize opportunities as they are presented. They also allow leveraging of the new technology and its treatment potential in messaging to patients about the level of care that can be provided.

To realize a return on any technology investment and maximize treatment options, dentists and their team members should be trained to make a difference, particularly by promoting and using the practice's new technology. Dentists should not try to do everything themselves, and efficient systems can help a practice hit targeted numbers and goals. Intelligent, sophisticated systems include scripting and support, which enable staff to educate patients about what services and treatments are available. However, because it is not enough to simply talk about dentistry, systems and technologies that foster a stronger practice/patient relationship inherently contribute to successful and confident integration.

This book, *Understanding, Assessing & Treating Dentomandibular Sensorimotor Dysfunction*, presents dentists and their team members with the scientific background, technology overview, and treatment implications of a complete system. The system assesses and addresses destructive force related dental problems, including headache pain. Germane to this discussion is an understanding of the evolution and application of technology in dental practice, as well as the necessity for a growing knowledge base. This base is focused on the neurophysiology of dental forces and its effects on the oral environment and health.

Chapter 1 succinctly reviews our profession's diagnostics and discoveries, as well as how they have contributed to dentistry's expanding role in our patient's health. It is that knowledge base that has broadened our understanding of the full impact of unbalanced or overloaded muscle forces, which are related to sensorimotor and somatosensory proprioceptive or nociceptive physiology. This is otherwise known as dentomandibular sensorimotor dysfunction. The role of this disorder, along with the spectrum of conditions and symptoms generally described by it, are thoroughly explained in Chapter 2.

In Chapter 3, readers begin to realize the role of dentistry in conservatively treating this disorder. The rationale for the development and use of the TruDenta system is detailed. Also, an outline of its systematic and objective assessment, monitoring, and therapeutic technology is provided. Chapter 4 reviews the manner in which the technology can be incorporated into dental practice to provide care for patients suffering with the symptoms of many types of dentomandibular sensorimotor dysfunction and force imbalances in the dental foundation.

In the book's final chapter, Chapter 5, the significance of providing patients with comprehensive and modern treatments is reinforced. This provision is achieved by using properly integrated technology that is inherently objective, therapeutic, and conservative. Overall, the text provides essential information to help the entire dental team wisely incorporate the new technology. It also establishes a clinical and medical reference for the necessity of treating the physiological causes of force related dental problems by following an objective approach to assessment, as well as providing straightforward and conservative care.

In closing, today's wonderful dental technologies can reinvigorate a dental practice with excitement and bring fresh perspectives to existing services. At a time when dentists and their team members are faced with simultaneously optimizing the potential of their practices and providing enhanced patient care, the right technological addition can also enable them to experience professional growth and personal satisfaction.

1 | Diagnostics, Discovery and Dentistry's Expanding Capabilities

Since the first mass produced toothbrush in the late 1700s, and moving into the 1800s with the introduction of modern toothpaste and dental floss, dentistry has evolved rapidly. The profession has experienced a proud history of innovatively applying research, technology, and proven techniques in order to address conditions and diseases affecting the oral cavity.[1] Today, both professionals and patients enjoy greater oral health, and the dental treatments they receive last longer and function more predictably. Many dentists are realizing a greater level of professional satisfaction due in part to providing a higher level of personalized care in an environment that recognizes the value of oral health. New and innovative technologies, as well as techniques enabling their application to oral

LEARNING OBJECTIVES

After reading this chapter, the reader should be able to:

1. Describe some of the technological innovations that have enhanced assessment and diagnosis of dental and oral conditions.

2. Discuss the impact of abnormal or unbalanced forces on the dental foundation.

3. Explain the anatomical, neurological, and physiological basis for dentists treating force related dental problems.

health, are contributing to such enhanced levels of patient care.

These technological innovations have, in many ways, transformed dentistry from a surgical profession into one emphasizing prevention and early intervention.[2] Prevention and early intervention, of course, are predicated on early and precise diagnostic information. The advent of technologically based diagnostic devices has enhanced the dentist's acuity for identifying oral diseases and, in some instances, their causes. By empowering dentists and oral healthcare providers to identify and manage oral diseases at the first signs, whether caries or oral cancer, diagnostic and treatment advances are improving and simplifying the interventions that are ultimately deemed necessary.

For example, the way in which caries are detected and managed today is no longer dependent upon visual assessment and traditional radiographs, but is instead based on diagnostics with greater sensitivity and specification. Devices including chairside tests of saliva, plaque, and biofilm, and bioluminescence, along with trans-illumination, laser fluorescence, and imaging, now enable dentists to detect the presence of disease at its earliest stages based on an understanding of the visual changes that represent the presence or risk of disease.[3-6] As a result, they now can prevent, arrest, reverse, and/or restore tooth structure faster, more minimally invasively, and more predictably.

Similarly, salivary diagnostics uses a saliva sample to identify, prevent, or evaluate risk factors for disease. Due to the fact that saliva's contents are an extraction of the cells found in the blood stream, the fluid represents the protein composition circulating throughout the body and whether it is healthy or diseased. Currently, salivary tests are being refined for identifying markers for diseases including breast and pancreatic cancer, cardiovascular disease, incipient infection, and diabetes mellitus.[7] Also, salivary diagnostics have relevance for detecting periodontal disease and its risk factors (e.g., inflammation), as well as HPV.[8]

Within the past decade, cytology-based DNA imaging tests and light technologies that have focused on the loss of autofluorescence also have begun to provide dentists with scientifically proven, chairside methods for the early screening and detection of oral cancer.[9] When the results of these technologically based diagnostic tools are combined with clinical assessment, oral healthcare providers can increase the evidence on which they base their decisions.

Likewise, cone beam computed tomography (CBCT) has been a valuable imaging tool for dentists in cases requiring three dimensional details, such as relating implant position to the mandibular canal, assessing impacted third molar root relationships, and planning orthognathic surgery. Additionally, CBCT has been beneficial in endodontics, particularly for identifying additional root canals in teeth that are not readily visible in conventional two dimensional images.[6] This technology may also reveal coincident conditions, including condylar pathologies and non-tooth-related abnormalities in the head and neck region.

■ Advancements in Understanding the Greater Dentomandibular Complex

Interestingly, it is this area—the greater head, neck, and dentofacial region—for which other technological and material science innovations have been introduced within the past 25 years for either diagnosing or treating oral-based problems. Numerous systems, such as high-strength ceramics or in-office CAD/CAM systems, respond to the need to restoratively resolve the effects of destructive conditions (e.g., wear, bruxism, tooth decay).[10-12] The need for developing such enhanced materials has been predicated on a clinical and research understanding of the effects of the oral environment on the longevity of restorations, as well as opposing natural dentition and the overall masticatory system.[13]

Other systems, such as cervical range of motion devices (CROM), or instrumental occlusal analysis equipment (T-Scan), offer insights into physiological and functional issues. These are issues that could be affecting the greater dentomandibular complex and/or contributing to related health problems in the greater head, neck, and dentofacial area (Figure 1.1).[14-18] Dentists have applied these technologies in everything ranging from diagnosis and planning to implant procedures. They have also been applied to determine restorative rehabilitations centering on occlusal adjustments. For example, with the availability of

The Dentomandibular Complex and Sensorimotor Dysfunction

Dentomandibular is a term used to collectively describe the mandible, upper three cervical vertebrae, and associated musculature that are related to the somatosensory and sensorimotor neurology surrounding the teeth and jaws via dendritic synapses that have developed within the trigeminal cervical nucleus (i.e., brainstem pathway).[24] This major neurological system of the brainstem mediates and controls afferent signals from the teeth to the trigeminal cervical nucleus, as well as carries information regarding headache, head and face pain, and neck pain to an individual's thalamus and on to the cortex. Approximately 40 percent of the afferent control into this column comes from the area around the teeth and jaws. Dentomandibular sensorimotor dysfunction, therefore, refers to force related and pain-related pathology, conditions, and symptoms originating in this area.[24]

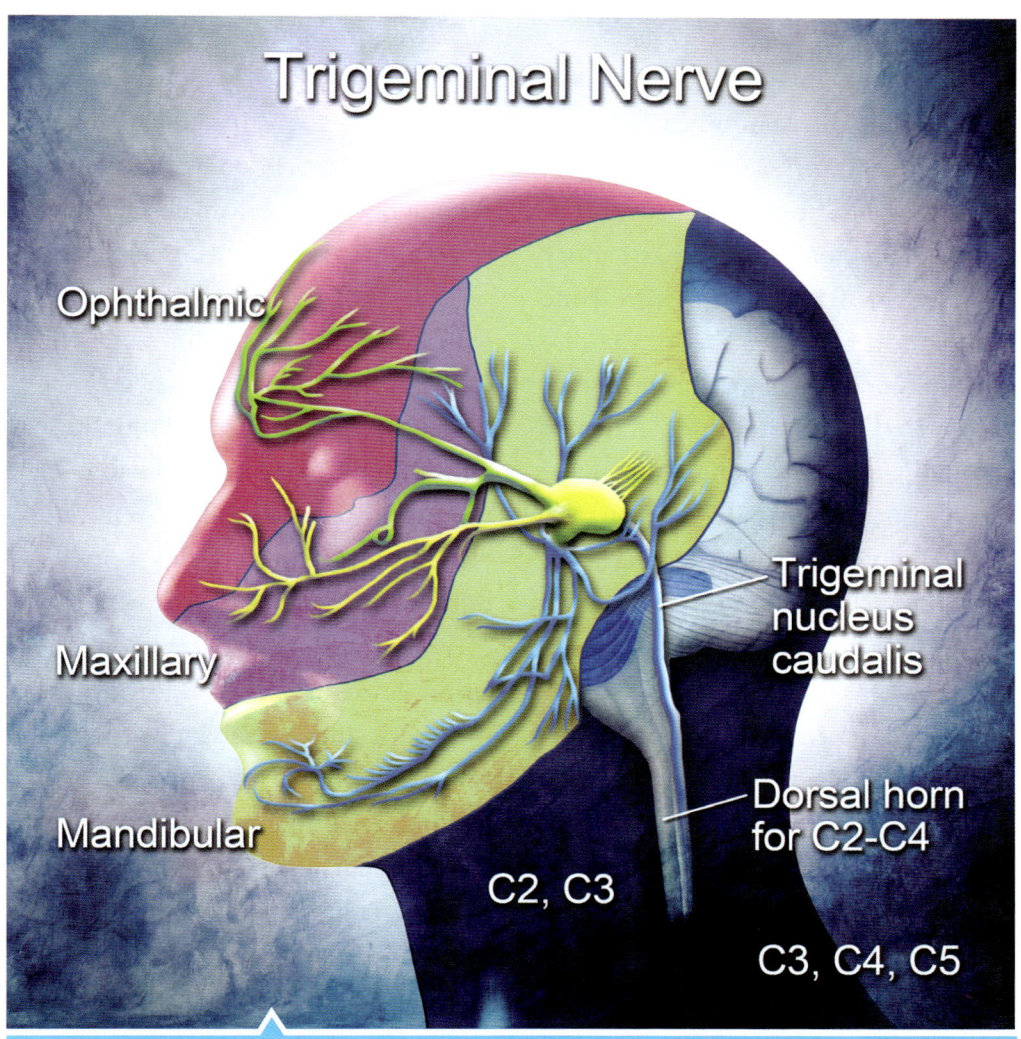

FIGURE 1.1. Dentomandibular sensorimotor dysfunction involves the mandible, upper three cervical vertebrae, and associated musculature that are related to the somatosensory and sensorimotor neurology surrounding the teeth and jaws via dendritic synapses that have developed within the trigeminal cervical nucleus (i.e., brainstem pathway).

electronic axiographic tracers, the movements of the condyles can be assessed, and magnetic resonance tomography imaging can be used to analyze the anatomical relation of the joint surfaces to the disk.[18] Additionally, pressure sensitive foils enable an analysis of masticatory forces, in conjunction with time resolution, in order to plot the distribution of forces within the occlusion.[15-17] The unifying objective of utilizing these assessment technologies is to provide patients with care that helps to establish long-term stability while also contributing to health.

These restorative and diagnostic approaches collectively recognize and reflect a greater knowledge and increasing understanding of the interrelationship between force overload and disease. They also acknowledge a better understanding of dysfunction within the oral environment, along with the masticatory system of which it is a part. Improper, un-balanced forces can result in open margins, fractures, abfractions, wear, sensitivity, mobility, or even failed restorations, all of which require treatment or retreatment.[19,20] In some instances, stronger and more durable all-ceramic restorations that can withstand the forces of mastication are necessary.

Symptoms and results of such diseases have collectively been addressed in restorative rehabilitations with an emphasis on occlusion. In the presence of a weak system and clenching/bruxing, occlusal instability contributes to the breakdown of natural tooth structure and restorative dentistry.[13,21] Regardless of the occlusal philosophy that is followed in order to complete restorations, recognizing the symptoms of malocclusion has been instrumental in helping to provide predictable, reliable, and long-lasting dental treatments.

Malocclusion refers to the interdigitation of the teeth or the location of teeth's centric stops that result in damage to the integrity of the tooth anatomy, periodontal interface, stomatognathic system as a whole, or pain. Abnormal forces between some or all teeth contribute to such an interdigitation. This definition allows a perspective on occlusion that addresses the direct relationship of functional physiology to observed and treated disease and degeneration.[22-24]

Pain resulting from the effects of malocclusion may manifest as hypersensitivity, deep tooth pain, jaw pain, or pain in the head and neck region that is served by the trigeminal cervical nucleus.[24-26] Therefore, it is understandable that the signs and symptoms of abnormal forces can involve the teeth, muscles, or joints (Figure 1.2). These combine to form the triad of anatomy which is referred to as the "dental foundation."[24] When abnormal forces affect the dental foundation, alterations and adaptations can occur to the masticatory musculature and the temporomandibular joint (TMJ), as well as the condyle and its ability to function.[24,27] In fact, malocclusion is just one of the many issues that can result from a disruption in the normal function of the musculature. As patients develop pathology or even suffer seemingly non-dental related trauma, changes can occur to the balance and function of the mandible. This can also occur when patients undergo dental treatments, whether they are restorations, orthodontics, or implant therapies. Changes in the dental foundation can be as simple as sore or sensitive teeth after restoration, or as complex as the creation of an adapted interdigitation to avoid extreme forces. Regardless, the patient's proprioceptive system is constantly changing. These changes may result in the dislocation of condyles during mastication, clenching, or early disk movement that often precedes disk displacement. Other results may include patterns of self-equilibration.[24,28-30]

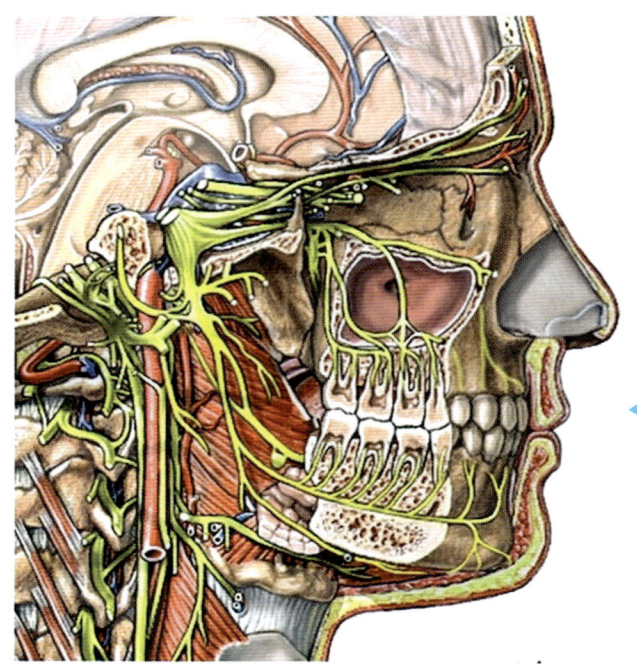

FIGURE 1.2.

The triad of anatomy that is referred to as the "dental foundation" is comprised of the teeth, muscles, and joints. Adaptive changes in any of these areas occasionally contribute to the conversion of acute pain to chronic pain. The sequelae of pain processes then lead to further neurochemical adaptations, as well as compensatory muscle activity that can result in myriad effects, such as damage to natural teeth or restorations, injury to periodontal structures, and pain.

Adaptive changes occasionally contribute to the conversion of acute pain to chronic pain. The sequelae of pain processes then lead to further neurochemical adaptations, as well as compensatory muscle activity that can result in a limited range of motion (e.g., mandibular or cervical) and/or trigger point muscle spasms.[30-32] Dentistry is clearly cognizant of the fact that an individual's dental occlusion must be addressed beyond the teeth. The presence of malocclusion, along with the forces contributing to it, affects the longevity of restorations, the joints, periodontal structures, head and neck muscles, function, and quality of life.[13,33]

The vast majority of dental related diseases can be categorized according to three primary issues (Table 1.1). Other restorative treatment may directly result from force related problems that originate from abnormal forces applied to the teeth by an individual's muscles. Therefore, the goal of modern occlusal-related treatments has been to balance the masticatory forces. This helps to prevent stress and dysfunction with the dental foundation and the dentomandibular area.[13,21,22,34]

To this end, a force-balanced occlusion is the objective when relieving individuals of occlusal dysfunction. A force-balanced occlusion is one defined as a normal or healthy occlusion in which the system of interdental forces is well distributed around the arch, with an unhindered path to closure and to mastication. A key aspect of relieving occlusal dysfunction is ensuring that the interdental forces are distributed down the long axis of the posterior teeth, so that the total forces are balanced in a 50/50, right/left ratio during a full closure to interdigitation. Additionally, during this process, the closure muscles should function with symmetry. There should also be musculoskeletal stability and symmetry of the TMJ condyles, while the disks are normally interposed at full closure.[13,35,36]

When the occlusion is force balanced, an individual is comfortable in rest and full closure. Their mandibular range of motion is within normal limits (e.g., 53 mm to 57 mm), and the individual does not experience acute or chronic pain. From a quality of life perspective, the person demonstrates normal posture, work abilities, and there are no dietary restrictions due to limitations of dental function.[13,24,37,38]

■ Opportunities Presented by Need and Knowledge

By combining technological innovations with clinical observation and evaluation, a greater understanding of the significance of muscle forces to occlusal problems, as well as the pain patients experience in the dentomandibular region, has been achieved.[35,36] Practical mea-

TABLE 1.1. Causes of Dental Disease[21]

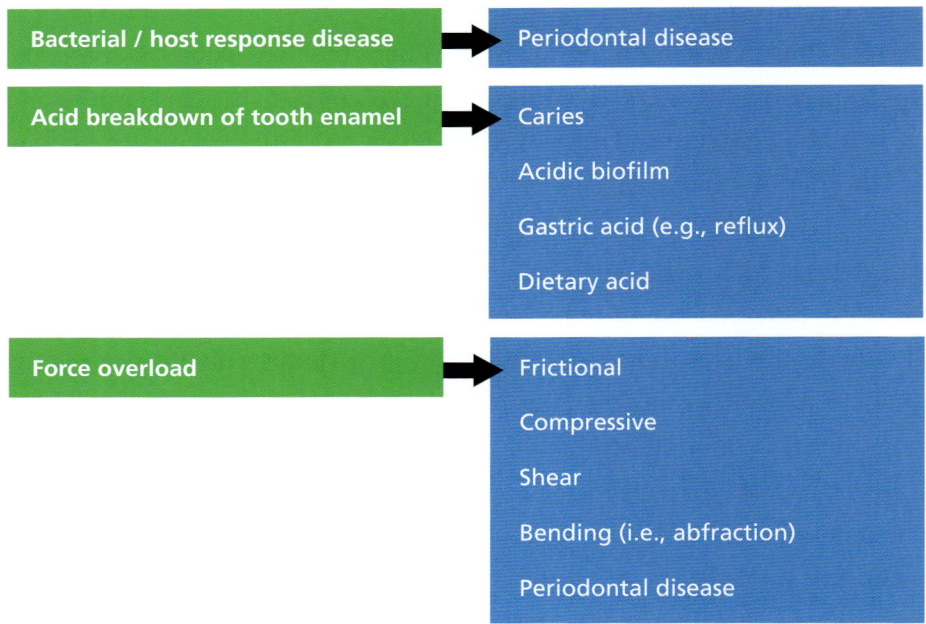

suring instruments have successfully identified occlusal interferences and heavier contacts (i.e., forces), along with muscle responses and pain symptoms that occur during masticatory function.[13,35,36] Technology has also demonstrated its utility in revealing significant discrepancies in jaw position and muscle function that contribute to chronic daily headaches.[39]

The availability of such objective data concerning pain stimuli in conjunction with masticatory function, combines with ongoing research into TMJ, orofacial, headache, and other systemic pain responses attributable to muscle forces. This combination of data and ongoing research has ushered another paradigm shift in the manner in which dentistry addresses patients who suffer from complex, sometimes debilitating discomfort issues.

For example, in the absence of definitive tissue pathology, greater emphasis has been placed on understanding that pain in some individuals may result from altered central nervous system pain processing. This particularly involves the masticatory muscles and soft tissues in the greater head and neck area.[40] Increased muscle tension and force, as associated with parafunctional habits and stress, are predictors of jaw and facial pain.[41] Additionally, headache is now partially explained by referred pain from myofacial trigger points in the posterior cervical, head, and shoulder muscles. It is in these areas in which peripheral mechanisms contribute to pericranial tenderness and the activation or sensitization of nociceptive nerve endings by liberating chemical mediators.[42]

Reversing parafunctional habits such as grinding, clenching, and bruxing through behavior modification has demonstrated promise in reducing the pain individuals experience from TMJ disorders (TMJ/D) and myofacial issues.[43,44] Among the pain conditions that dentists may encounter are TMJ/D, neuropathic pain disorders, and headaches, whether they are common, chronic, or migraine. Deprogrammers have been part of the process of "educating" or "re-training" the masticatory muscles, acknowledging the muscles' role in the forces contributing to pain. They also acknowledge the fact that controlling the perpetuating factors (i.e., force) can help control, reduce, or eliminate pain.[44,45] In fact, muscle hyperactivity is a known potential source of symptomatology in individuals with TMJ/D and other dentomandibular-related pain, since it creates a feedback mechanism involving the trigeminal nerve.[46]

Interestingly, it is the interrelation of the muscles of mastication, the trigeminal nerve, and the effect of force on this complex that places the assessment and therapeutic rehabilitation of patients suffering with headache and dental-related pain within the realm of dentistry.[47] According to the American Dental Association, dentists' expertise lies not only in treating the teeth and gingival tissues, but also in caring for the muscles of the head, neck, and jaw, as well as the nervous system of the head, neck, and other areas.[48]

In particular, the tight connections that the trigeminal nerve pathways have with all head and neck nociceptive neurology comprise the primary neural afferent and efferent system of the dentomandibular region.[47] Research into neurophysiology and neuroplasticity further suggests the dentist's role in assisting with normal neurological function, including pain control, by managing normal function in the head and neck. This, of course, encompasses normal mastication, airway management, normal deglutition, normal expression, and especially normal force balance via the proprioceptive and somatosensory systems.[49]

Therefore, any patient with problems based in the teeth, muscles, or joints or in the trigeminal cervical nucleus should be cared for by a knowledgeable dentist in order to realize the greatest opportunity for pain resolution.[47-49] Other medical professionals who treat some of these "foundation" problems can achieve short-term success because they are not addressing, nor can they control, the afferent signals from the teeth to the trigeminal cervical nucleus. This brainstem pathway conducts all the information regarding headache, head and face pain, and TMJ/D related pain to the patient's thalamus and on to the cortex. Approximately 40 percent of the afferent control into this pathway originates from the dentomandibular area surrounding the teeth and jaws.[47,49]

The number of patients suffering from pain and discomfort that originates in this area is staggering. According to the National Headache Foundation, more than 29 million Americans suffer from migraines. The causes include trigger factors such as dietary factors, hormonal variations, sleep disorders, and others that excite brain cells and ultimately trigger a reaction in the trigeminal nerve, resulting in pain.[50] Individuals suffering with migraines lose more than 157 million work and school days each year due to pain.[51] In addition to migraine sufferers, an estimated 90 percent of the population suffers from headaches.[51]

Dentists themselves are all too aware of the increasing numbers of patients suffering with TMJ/D issues. The National Institute of Dental and Craniofacial Research (NIDCR) estimates that more than 10 million Americans suffer from TMJ/D, but the number could actually fall between a total of 15 and 45 million patients with some type of TMJ issue.[52]

■ The Time Is Now

Unquestionably, treatments for TMJ/D, pain, and dysfunction have evolved over the years. This is due to diagnostics, clinical findings, and new therapeutic regimens that enable dentists to relieve patients' suffering.[53] However, with the increasing understanding of the mechanisms that exacerbate and/or cause pain in the face, head, oral environment, and the joints and muscles in these areas, now is the time for dentistry to embrace a new paradigm in the assessment, rehabilitation, and treatment of destructive force related dental problems.

For years, dentists and their staff have often been the first line of defense and intervention for their patients. This has become increasingly so, as the association between oral and systemic diseases has taken center stage in dentistry and medicine. Whether based on suspicions and clinical findings indicating sleep disordered breathing, snoring, uncontrolled diabetes that correlates to periodontal pathogens, or eating disorders reflected in lingual tooth wear and erosion, dentists have helped to manage the overall health and well-being of their patients, as well as serve as a professional resource for dental-related therapies.[54,55]

Just as dentistry has moved into the realm of oral systemic care as a collaborative partner with its physician colleagues in medicine, now is the time for dentistry to embrace dental headache care. It is also time for dentistry to provide relief and therapy for pain symptoms associated with the greater head, neck, and dentofacial area.[56] With the research and technology that has been developed for, and proven effective in, other disciplines, including sports medicine and rehabilitation, dentists are now well positioned to address the patient population that suffers with the debilitating symptoms of dentomandibular sensorimotor dysfunction.

References

1. DiMatteo AM. Dental inventors and the greatest innovations in dental history. *Inside Dentistry*. May 2009:88-102.

2. DiMatteo AM. Dentistry: Did you choose the right profession? *Inside Dentistry*. Nov/Dec 2006:52-59.

3. Twetman S, Axelsson S, Dahlén G, Espelid I, Mejàre I, Norlund A, Tranæus S. Adjunct methods for caries detection: A systematic review of literature. *Acta Odontol Scand*. 2012 May 28. [Epub ahead of print]

4. Karlsson L. Caries detection methods based on changes in optical properties between healthy and carious tissue. *Int J Dent*. 2010;2010:270729. [Epub 2010 Mar 28]

5. Strassler HE, Sensi LG. Technology-enhanced caries detection and diagnosis. *Compend Contin Educ Dent*. 2008 Oct;29(8):464-5, 468, 470 passim.

6. Pette GA, Norkin FJ, Ganeles J, Hardigan P, Lask E, Zfaz S, Parker W. Incidental findings from a retrospective study of 318 cone beam computed tomography consultation reports. *Int J Oral Maxillofac Implants*. 2012 May-Jun;27(3):595-603.

7. Brinkmann O, Spielmann N, Wong DT. Salivary diagnostics: moving to the next level. *Dent Today*. 2012 Jun;31(6):54, 56-7; quiz 58-9.

8. Giannobile WV, McDevitt JT, Niedbala RS, Malamud D. Translational and clinical applications of salivary diagnostics. *Adv Dent Res*. 2011 Oct;23(4):375-80.

9. Palmer O, Grannum R. Oral cancer detection. *Dent Clin North Am*. 2011 Jul;55(3):537-48, viii-ix.

10. Tysowsky GW. The science behind lithium disilicate: a metal-free alternative. *Dent Today*. 2009 Mar;28(3):112-3.

11. Strub JR, Rekow ED, Witkowski S. Computer-aided design and fabrication of dental restorations: current systems and future possibilities. *J Am Dent Assoc*. 2006 Sep;137(9):1289-96.

12. Kugel G. Materials continue to expand dentistry's options. *Compend Contin Educ Dent*. 2012 Jan;33(1):80.

13. Dawson P. *Functional Occlusion: From TMJ to Smile Design*. Canada: Mosby, Inc.; 2007.

14. Ogince M, Hall T, Robinson K, Blackmore AM. The diagnostic validity of the cervical flexion-rotation test in C1/2-related cervicogenic headache. *Man Ther*. 2007 Aug;12(3):256-62.

15. Garg AK. Analyzing dental occlusion for implants: Tekscan's TScan III. *Dent Implantol Update*. 2007 Sep; 18(9):65-70.

16. Koos B, Godt A, Schille C, Göz G. Precision of an instrumentation-based method of analyzing occlusion and its resulting distribution of forces in the dental arch. *J Orofac Orthop.* 2010 Nov; 71(6):403-10.

17. Koos B, Holler J, Schille C, Godt A. Time-dependent analysis and representation of force distribution and occlusion contact in the masticatory cycle. *J Orofac Orthop.* 2012 May; 73(3):204-14.

18. Tymofiyeva O, Proff P, Richter EJ, Jakob P, Fanghanel J, Gedrange T, Rottner K. Correlation of MRT imaging with real-time axiography of TMJ clicks. *Ann Anat.* 2007;189(4):356-61.

19. Simon J. Biomechanically-induced dental disease. *Gen Dent.* 2000 Sep-Oct;48(5):598-605.

20. Francisconi LF, Graeff MS, Martins Lde M, Franco EB, Mondelli RF, Francisconi PA, Pereira JC. The effects of occlusal loading on the margins of cervical restorations. *J Am Dent Assoc.* 2009 Oct;140(10):1275-82.

21. Hess LA. The relevance of occlusion in the golden age of esthetics. *Inside Dent.* 2008:38-44.

22. McNeill C. Occlusion: what it is and what it is not. *J Calif Dent Assoc.* 2000 Oct;28(10):748-58.

23. Mackie A, Lyons K. The role of occlusion in temporomandibular disorders--a review of the literature. *N Z Dent J.* 2008 Jun;104(2):54-9.

24. Montgomery MW, Shuman L, Morgan A. T-scan dental force analysis for routine dental examination. *Dent Today*. 2011 Jul;30(7):112-4, 116.

25. Frisardi G, Chessa G, Sau G, Frisardi F. Trigeminal electrophysiology: a 2x2 matrix model for differential diagnosis between temporomandibular disorders and orofacial pain. *BMC Musculoskelet Disord*. 2010 Jul 1; 11:141.

26. Hegarty AM, Zakrzewska JM. Differential diagnosis for orofacial pain, including sinusitis, TMD, trigeminal neuralgia. *Dent Update*. 2011 Jul-Aug;38(6):396-400, 402-3, 405-6 passim.

27. Okeson JP. Occlusion, condylar position and TMD: Where is the controversy? Where is the evidence. Lecture. 148th American Dental Association Annual Session; September 28, 2007: San Francisco, CA.

28. Schindler HJ, Rues S, Türp JC, Schweizerhof K, Lenz J. Jaw clenching: muscle and joint forces, optimization strategies. *J Dent Res*. 2007 Sep;86(9):843-7.

29. Kampe T. Function and dysfunction of the masticatory system in individuals with intact and restored dentitions. A clinical, psychological and physiological study. *Swed Dent J Suppl*. 1987;42:1-68.

30. Lodetti G, Mapelli A, Musto F, Rosati R, Sforza C. EMG spectral characteristics of masticatory muscles and upper trapezius during maximum voluntary teeth clenching. *J Electromyogr Kinesiol*. 2012 Feb;22(1):103-9. [Epub 2011 Nov 17]

31. Ohrbach R, Fillingim RB, Mulkey F, Gonzalez Y, Gordon S, Gremillion H, Lim PF, Ribeiro-Dasilva M, Greenspan JD, Knott C, Maixner W, Slade G. Clinical findings and pain symptoms as potential risk factors for chronic TMD: descriptive data and empirically identified domains from the OPPERA case-control study. *J Pain*. 2011 Nov;12(11 Suppl):T27-45.

32. Fernandez-de-Las-Penas C, Ge HY, Alonso-Blanco C, Gonzalez-Iglesias J, Arendt-Nielson L. Referred pain areas of active myofascial trigger points in head, neck, and shoulder muscles, in chronic tension type headache. *J Body Mov Ther*. 2010 Oct;14(4):391-6.

33. Velly AM, Look JO, Carlson C, Lenton PA, Kang W, Holcroft CA, Fricton JR. The effect of catastrophizing and depression on chronic pain--a prospective cohort study of temporomandibular muscle and joint pain disorders. *Pain*. 2011 Oct;152(10):2377-83.

34. Ackerman JL, Ackerman MB, Kean MR. A Philadelphia fable: how ideal occlusion became the philosopher's stone of orthodontics. *Angle Orthod*. 2007; 77(1):192-194.

35. Maness WL. Force movie. A time and force view of occlusion. *Compend Contin Educ Dent*. 1989;10:404-8.

36. Kerstein RB. Treatment of myofacial pain dysfunction syndrome with occlusal therapy to reduce lengthy disclusion time—a recall study. *J Craniomandib Pract*. 1995;13(2):105-15.

37. Okeson JP. *Management of Temporomandibular Disorders and Occlusion*, 6th Edition. Mosby: 2008.

38. Wright EF. *Manual of Temporomandibular Disorders*. 2nd Edition. Wiley:Blackwell:2009.

39. Didier H, Marchetti C, Borromeo G, Tullo V, D'amico D, Bussone G, Santoro F. Chronic daily headache: suggestion for the neuromuscular oral therapy. *Neurol Sci*. 2011 May;32 Suppl 1; S161-4.

40. Cairns BE. Pathophysiology of TMD pain—basic mechanisms and their implications for pharmacotherapy. *J Oral Rehabil*. 2010 May; 37(6):391-410.

41. Glaros AG, Williams K, Lausten L. The role of parafunctions, emotions and stress in predicting facial pain. *J Am Dent Assoc*. 2005 Apr; 136(4):451-8.

42. Fernandez-de-las-Penas C, Cuadrado ML, Arendt-Nielson L, Simons DG, Pareja JA. Myofascial trigger points and sensitization: an updated pain model for tension-type headache. *Cephalalgia*. 2007 May;27(5):383-93. Epub 2007 May 14.

43. Glaros AG. Temporomandibular disorders and facial pain: a psychophysiological perspective. *Appl Psycholphysiol Biofeedback*. 2008 Sep;33(3):161-171.

44. Okeson JP, deLeeuw R. Differential diagnosis of temporomandibular disorders and other orofacial pain disorders. *Dent Clin North Am*. 2011 Jan;55(1):105-20.

45. McKee JR. Comparing condylar positions achieved through bimanual manipulation to condylar positions achieved through masticatory muscle contraction against an anterior deprogrammer: a pilot study. *J Prosthet Dent*. 2005 Oct;94(4):389-93.

46. Kerstein RB. Reducing chronic masseter and temporalis muscular hyperactivity with computer-guided occlusal adjustments. *Compend Contin Educ Dent*. 2010 Sep;31(7):530-4, 536, 538.

47. Bogduk N. The neck and headaches. *Neurol Clin*. 2004 Feb;22(1):151-71, vii.

48. American Dental Association. Dentists: Doctors of Oral Health. http://www.ada.org/4504.aspx. Accessed July 3, 2012.

49. Sessle BJ. Mechanisms of oral somatosensory and motor functions and their clinical correlates. *J Oral Rehabil*. 2006 Apr. 33(4):243-61.

50. National Headache Foundation. http://www.headaches.org/education/Headache_Topic_Sheets/Migraine. Accessed July 3, 2012.

51. Headache. *US News and World Report*. 2006. http://health.usnews.com/health-conditions/brain-health/headache. Accessed July 3, 2012.

52. National Institute of Dental and Craniofacial Research. http://www.nidcr.nih.gov/DataStatistics/ByPopulation/Adults/

53. Dym H, Israel H. Diagnosis and treatment of temporomandibular disorders. *Dent Clin North Am*. 2012 Jan;56(1):49-61.

54. Mohsenin N, Mostofi MT, Mohsenin V. The role of oral appliances in treating obstructive sleep apnea. *J Am Dent Assoc.* 2003 Apr;134(4):442-9.

55. Ashcroft A, Milosevic A. The eating disorders: 2. Behavioral and dental management. *Dent Update.* 2007 Dec;34(10):612-6, 619-20.

56. Fricton JR, Okeson JP. Broad support evident for the emerging specialty of orofacial pain. *Tex Dent J.* 2000 Jul; 117(7):22-5.

Chapter 1 Self-Assessment Quiz

1. Approximately 40 percent of the afferent control into the trigeminal cervical nucleus originates from the area surrounding the teeth and jaws.

    a. True.

    b. False.

2. Which of the following is not an indication that an individual's occlusion is force balanced?

    a. They are comfortable in rest and full closure.

    b. Their mandibular range of motion is within normal limits.

    c. They experience acute or chronic pain.

    d. All of the above.

(cont.)

Chapter 1 Self-Assessment Quiz (cont.)

3. Balancing the masticatory forces helps to achieve which of the following?

   a. Prevent stress within the dental foundation.

   b. Prevent dysfunction within the dentomandibular area.

   c. Distribute dental forces down the long axis of posterior teeth in a 50/50 right/left ratio.

   d. All of the above.

4. Adaptive changes in the dentomandibular area can result in which of the following?

   a. Conversion of acute pain to chronic pain.

   b. Limited mandibular range of motion.

   c. Both a and b.

   d. None of the above.

(cont.)

Chapter 1 Self-Assessment Quiz (cont.)

5. Headache can no longer be partially explained by referred pain from myofacial trigger points.

    a. True.
    b. False.

2 | Dentomandibular Sensorimotor Dysfunction and Its Role in Chronic Pain

Dentomandibular sensorimotor dysfunction describes conditions and physiology that are related to the stimulus and response that take place in the orofacial area, head, and neck via applied neurology and musculature linked by the trigeminal cervical nucleus.[1-3] The disorder involves the temporomandibular joints (TMJs), masticatory musculature, jaw function, dental forces, and the common neurology of these structures and functions. Dentomandibular sensorimotor dysfunction can generally involve a spectrum of conditions and symptoms (Table 2.1).

The common element in all of these conditions is the effect of unbalanced or overloaded muscle forces related to sensorimotor and so-

> **LEARNING OBJECTIVES**
>
> After reading this chapter, the reader should be able to:
>
> 1. Describe the symptoms and conditions associated with dentomandibular sensorimotor dysfunction.
>
> 2. Discuss the musculature and central neurology involved with dentomandibular sensorimotor dysfunction.
>
> 3. Describe the rationale for a progressive approach to rehabilitating the tissues in the dentomandibular area as a means to balance the dental foundation and relieve pain.

TABLE 2.1. Conditions and Symptoms Generally Described as Dentomandibular Sensorimotor Dysfunction[3]

Headache/migraine	Clenching with or without torus formation
Myofacial pain	Bruxism
Tinnitus	Tooth wear
TMJ disorders	Abfractions
Pulpitis	Tooth fracture/damage
Poor airway control	Restricted range of motion and postural adaptations
Central nervous system changes in brain chemistry and neurotransmitter balance	Unstable dental arch form
Sleep/arousal disorders	

matosensory proprioceptive or nociceptive physiology.[1-3] Characterized by the forces generated by the muscles in this area (Figure 2.1), dentomandibular sensorimotor dysfunction results from the abnormal forces that cause an unbalanced dental foundation. Similarly, reflex proprioception results in dysfunction, as do injury and pain.[4] Dysfunction then contributes to further damage or disability. The dental foundation is considered to be out of balance when any of several conditions exist (Table 2.2).

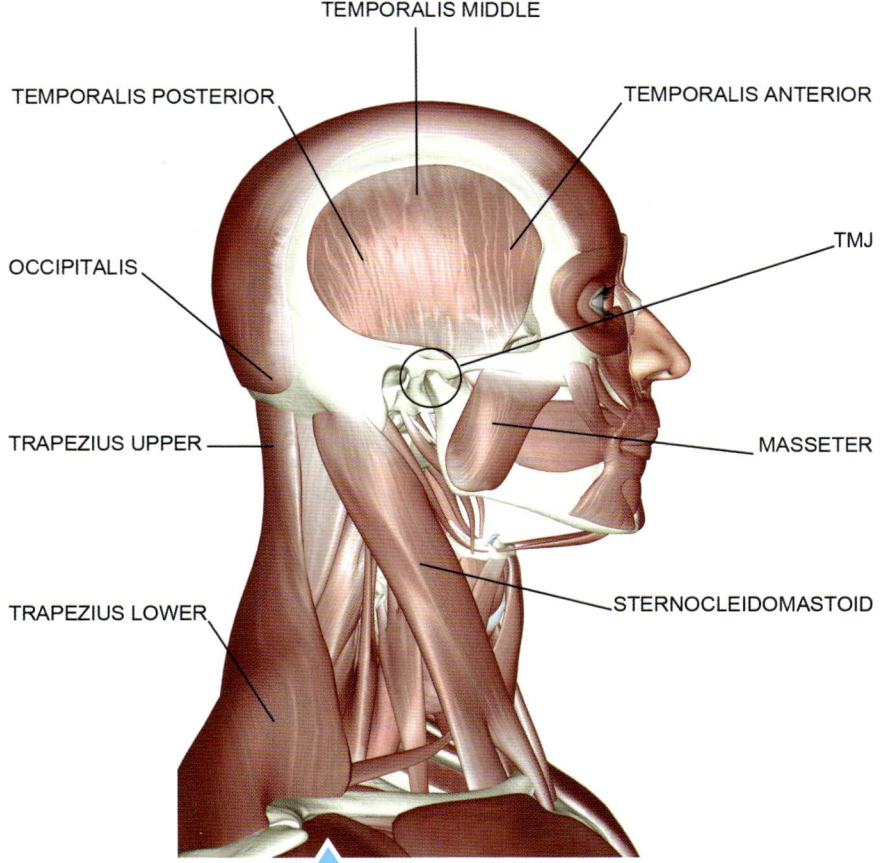

FIGURE 2.1. The effect of unbalanced or overloaded muscle forces related to sensorimotor and somatosensory proprioceptive or nociceptive physiology is the common element in conditions related to dentomandibular sensorimotor dysfunction.

Clinically managing these problems relies on controlling pain and inflammation. It also relies upon rehabilitating the system to normal function and range of motion, as well as orthopedic, orthodontic, and dental stabilization of the stomatognathic system. However, doing so is predicated on a solid understanding of the anatomy and physiology

TABLE 2.2. Conditions Indicating an Unbalanced System

- Accelerated aging or degeneration of the temporomandibular condyles
- Temporomandibular joint vibrations indicative of disk movement, disk derangement, or inflammation
- Tooth damage or degeneration related to abnormal forces
- Limited range of motion of the mandible or the cervical spine
- Presence of sore or painful muscles of the head and neck, especially the presence of "trigger points"
- Symptoms of pain that emanate from the structures connected via and controlled by the trigeminal cervical nucleus, especially headache
- Any lifestyle disability related to the teeth, muscles, or joints of the head and neck
- Abnormal forces are detected in the dentition by examination
- Injuries have occurred that affect any of the above structures or activities

of the head and neck. This is then combined with addressing a patient's dental treatment issues.[5] For many reasons, dentists have traditionally isolated the teeth and their pathology from the functional and parafunctional physiology that can cause wear, damage, fracture, abfractions, failure of restorations, and pain for their patients. These traumas and degenerations are only the signs and symptoms of the force related, underlying problem.

The nexus of tooth related problems, in relation to musculoskeletal

TABLE 2.3. Components of the Dentomandibular Sensorimotor Complex

Anatomical/ Neurological Structure	Function	Characteristics
Masseter	The masseter muscles are jaw muscles whose name is derived from the Greek word "to chew." A major muscle of mastication, its primary action and function is elevating and protracting the mandible. Located on each side of the face at the back of the jaw, these muscles are easily visible or palpable when the jaw is clenched, since they contract strongly just in front of the lower ears.	The superficial portion inserts on the ramus of the mandible, and the deep portion inserts on the upper half of the ramus and the lateral surface of the coronoid process of the mandible. Despite its size, masseter muscles are among the strongest. The average human can bite down with a force of 150 pounds, and bites of more than 250 pounds are within normal limits.
Lateral Pterygoid	The lateral pterygoid muscles (i.e., right and left) together protract (or protrude) and depress the mandible, as well as individually move the mandible from side to side. In combination with the digastric muscle, it is also responsible for opening the lower jaw during the translation phase of opening. The lateral pterygoid inserts at the condyle of the mandible and temporomandibular joint between 50 and 60 percent of the time.	Shaped like a partially unfolded fan, the lateral pterygoid has two bellies. The upper belly of the lateral pterygoid attaches primarily to the articular disk (between 50 and 60 percent of the time), while the lower belly attaches to the neck of the condyle. The two bellies may work independently, but usually in concert to maintain the articular disk's position at the closest point of contract between the condyle and the glenoid fossa during both the rotational phase of jaw opening and the translational phase. In pathologic conditions, the two bellies can contract at different rates, causing the articular disk to be pulled ahead of the condyle during translation. This can tear the cartilage, damaging the joint and allow the condyle to snap against the glenoid fossa, resulting in the clicking that temporomandibular joint disorder (TMJ/D) patients notice when opening or closing their mouths.

(cont.)

TABLE 2.3. Components of the Dentomandibular Sensorimotor Complex

Anatomical/ Neurological Structure	Function	Characteristics
Medial Pterygoid	The masseter and medial pterygoid function like a contractile "hammock" in which the lower jaw rests. These two muscles are more or less "twins", with the masseter acting on the outside of the lower jaw and the medial pterygoid on the inside. Together they clench, but do not make lateral movements. They are primarily affected in an imbalance of the vertical dimension of occlusion.	The medial pterygoid muscle arises from the medial surfaces of the lateral pterygoid plate, which is attached to the undersurface of the temporal bone. In other words, it is attached to the undersurface of the skull, just behind the last upper tooth. The medial pterygoid fibers are directed downward and backward, similar to the masseter, but on the inside of the mandible. The muscle inserts to the inside of the lower border and angle of the mandible.
Temporomandibular Joint Capsule	The temporomandibular joint capsule attaches to the articular eminence, the articular disk, and the neck of the mandibular condyle.	The temporomandibular joint capsule is a fibrous membrane surrounding the joint, incorporating the articular eminence.
Temporalis	The temporalis is a muscle of mastication, and its role is similar to the masseter (i.e., to elevate the mandible and close the mouth), but its horizontal fibers in the posterior part of the muscle also retract the mandible.	The temporalis muscle is a large, thin, fan-shaped muscle located on the inside of the skull, above and in front of the ear. It inserts at the coronoid process and anterior ramus of the mandible, passing down beneath the zygomatic arch.

(cont.)

TABLE 2.3. Components of the Dentomandibular Sensorimotor Complex

Anatomical/ Neurological Structure	Function	Characteristics
Digastrics	The digastric assists the lateral pterygoid in depressing the mandible and opening the jaw, primarily during maximum depression or very quick, forceful mouth opening. It also elevates the hyoid bone.	The digastric is a double muscle of the throat, one for each side of the jaw and neck, located under the chin, behind and below the corner of the jaw, and immediately in front of the top of the sternocleidomastoid. Its name is derived from the Greek word for "two bellies." The digastric is comprised of anterior and posterior bellies. The anterior belly extends from the digastric fossa of the mandible, while the posterior belly extends from the mastoid notch of the temporal bone. Both then insert to the body of the hyoid bone via a fibrous loop over a common intermediate tendon between the two bellies. The digastrics can become overworked from the pressure of an overactive masseter accompanied by habitual open mouth breathing due to sinus problems, secondary to bruxism, or while sleeping (e.g., sleep disorders).
Suboccipitals	The suboccipital muscles extend the head and rotate it toward the same side.	Suboccipital muscles are located on the underside of the occipital bone and include the rectus capitis posterior major, rectus capitis posterior minor, obliquus capitis inferior, and obliquus capitis superior. The rectus capitis posterior minor muscle extends from the middle of the posterior arch of the atlas to the occipit. The rectus capitis posterior major extends from the spinous process of the atlas to the occipital bone, lateral to the site of insertion of the rectus capitis posterior minor. The obliquus capitis inferior muscle extends from the spine of the axis vertebra to the transverse process of the atlas. The obliquus capitis superior muscle extends from the transverse process of the atlas to the occiput.

(cont.)

TABLE 2.3. Components of the Dentomandibular Sensorimotor Complex

Anatomical/ Neurological Structure	Function	Characteristics
Sternocleidomastoid	The right side of the sternocleidomastoid rotates the head to the left and flexes it to the right. The left side rotates the head to the right and flexes it to the left. Both sides together flex the neck and head forward. This muscle also is an important accessory muscle of respiratory inhalation and is highly active during high chest breathing, especially during rapid breathing.	The sternocleidomastoid is a muscle of the neck so-named because it originates at the sternum and clavicle, extending diagonally across the front and side of the neck, inserting on the mastoid process that is an easily located bony prominence behind the ear. This two sided muscle is large and ropy, making it the most prominent muscle visible at the front of the neck.
Upper Trapezius	The upper trapezius fibers work synergistically with the sternocleidomastoid in head and neck movements, but primarily function to elevate and adduct the shoulder girdle, as well as extend the head.	Although usually discussed as one muscle, the trapezius is separated into distinct groups of fibers that run in different directions and, therefore, have slightly different movement roles. These different fiber groups are usually referred to as the upper, middle, and lower trapezius. The trapezius extends from the base of the skull to the lower thoracic spine, and laterally from the clavicle to the entire length of the spine of scapula. The muscle derives its name from the diamond or kite-shaped trapezoid formed by two of the trapezii muscle fibers.
Condyle	The condyle is the jaw joint component responsible for movement in two directions.	The condyle is the slightly rounded end of the mandible that fits loosely into an elliptical cavity on the maxilla.
Protective Disk	The protective disk prevents the jaw bones from rubbing together.	

(cont.)

TABLE 2.3 Components of the Dentomandibular Sensorimotor Complex

Anatomical/ Neurological Structure	Function	Characteristics
Posterior Ligament	The posterior ligament prevents the disk from dislocating by serving as a band that pulls the disk back into position when the jaw closes.	
Brachial Arch Cranial Nerves	Brachial arch cranial nerves communicate and interact with each other through the brain stem, controlling the jaw, face, neck, shoulders, and other areas of the greater dentomandibular region.	The brachial arch cranial nerves sit in the lateral or back column of the brain stem. The jaw is controlled by the CN 5 nerve, the face by the CN 7, and the neck and shoulder by the CN 11.
Trigeminal Nerve	Communicate afferent and sensory information to the head, shoulder, neck, and facial areas, including the dentomandibular region.	The trigeminal nerve is the largest and most complex of the cranial nerves.
Glia	Glia cells support and protect neurons, as well as provide nutrients and oxygen to neurons.	Glia are non-neuronal cells that contribute to signal transmission in the nervous system.

and neurological physiology, is the point where forces are applied to the teeth or a bolus of food in a way that develops and determines the patterns of muscle activity through the sensorimotor neurology via the brainstem. The forces between the teeth via the musculature are altered when various circumstances occur. They are altered when neurology is abnormal (e.g., chronic pain). They can also be altered when muscle patterns are driven by central nervous system requirements (e.g., parafunction during sleep disturbances), or when the proprioception of the teeth is altered (e.g., sensitization or restorative changes).[6-9]

■ *Musculature and Joint Considerations*

In order for dentists to better interpret how the normal function of the sensorimotor apparatus will assist in relieving, reversing, or re-establishing health in a patient with dentomandibular sensorimotor dysfunction, they must understand the cranial and cervical nerves that serve the area, related musculature, and the central neurology of the trigeminal cervical nucleus (Table 2.3).[1-3] This paradigm shift in the thought processes for assessing and subsequently treating force related conditions that result in dental problems and chronic head and neck pain inherently leads to rehabilitation, therapy, and treatment. All of this is designed to resolve the issues in a healthy and balanced manner.

During mastication (Figures 2.2 through 2.5), the jaw opens and the first movement of the condyle in open position is downward. The TMJ is a ginglymo-arthrodial joint. A ginglymus joint is a hinge joint, and an arthrodia joint is a gliding joint. The TMJ is the only joint that both hinges and glides. It does not rotate in a static hinge position, but essentially has a multifocal axis whereby the axis focal position is constantly changing upon every movement of the jaw. These are termed instantaneous centers of rotation.

Dentomandibular Sensorimotor Dysfunction and Its Role in Chronic Pain

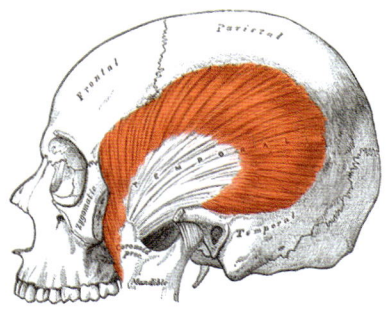

FIGURE 2.2. The temporalis muscle is innervated by the mandibular nerve CN V (V-3). It originates in the temporal lines on the parietal bone of the skull.

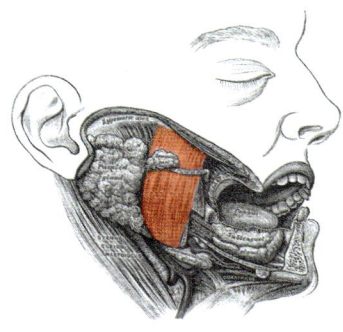

FIGURE 2.3. The temporal mandibular joint capsule is innervated by the auriculotemporal and massetric branches of the mandibular branch of the trigeminal nerve (i.e., CN V (V-3)).

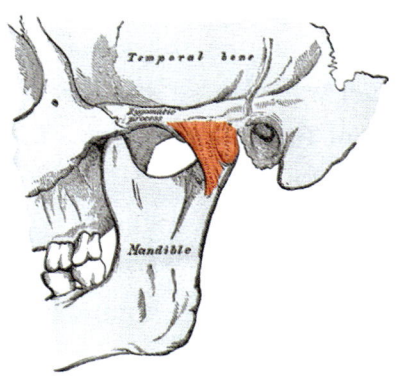

FIGURE 2.4. The masseter muscle originates in the zygomatic arch and maxilla. It is innervated by the mandibular nerve CN V (V3). It is palpated by squeezing the cheek on the inside of the mouth with five pounds of pressure to locate any tight bands or trigger points that may be in the muscle.

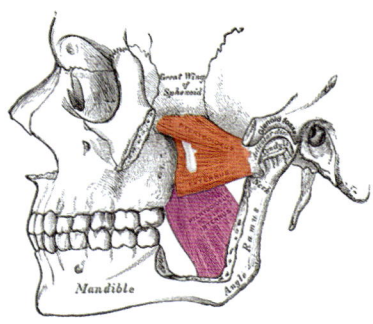

FIGURE 2.5. The lateral pterygoid muscle is innervated by the mandibular nerve CN V(V-3). It is palpated by placing the forefinger over the buccal area of the maxillary third molar region and exerting pressure in a posterior, superior, and medial direction, then applying three pounds of pressure.

There is one consistent factor to the TMJ upon opening. The first movement of the jaw upon opening is always a downward movement.

A critical component of this process is the mandibular condylar cartilage, which helps to facilitate articulation with the TMJ disk, while also reducing loads on the underlying bone.[10] All teeth should touch at the same time that the lower jaw follows the arc of closure, thus distributing the forces in a balanced way and preventing activation of the muscles. In other words, the system is at rest and stress-free.[5-7]

However, the medial pterygoid muscle is most heavily loaded during clenching, and the accentuated horizontal force provokes the highest loading within the medial and lateral pterygoids.[11,12] Dental symptoms caused by clenching and grinding include wear and restorative failure, among other symptoms. Research has demonstrated that individuals with restored dentition demonstrate more parafunctional activity and higher levels of muscular tension.[13]

Muscle hyperactivity is a known factor leading to increased and abnormal force that is degenerative, destructive, and painful. An increased volume of periodontal ligament compressions creates additive and excessive functional muscle contractions via a feedback mechanism involving the trigeminal nerve.[14]

■ *Neurophysiological Considerations*

The role of the trigeminal nerve, which is the largest and most complex of the cranial nerves, in orofacial pain and TMJ disorders (TMJ/D) is well recognized.[15] Even the first and smallest division (i.e., ophthalmic), which is purely sensory and afferent in function, may be implicated in orofacial pain.[16] The maxillary, or second, division of the trigeminal nerve provides sensory communication to all structures in and around the maxillary bone and midfacial region. This includes—but is not limited to—the soft palate, maxillary gingiva, upper lip, roof of the mouth, and maxillary teeth.[17] This complex division of the trigeminal nerve is closely linked to orofacial pain. However, the largest division of the trigeminal nerve, the mandibular or third division, is considered a mixed nerve that conveys afferent fibers, as well as efferent fibers, to the masticatory muscles (i.e., mylohyoid and anterior digastric muscles) and others.[18] Intimately linked with dentistry, this complicated division of the trigeminal nerve refers pain to other areas within its branches, as well as to other trigeminal divisions, such as the maxilla. It is this pathway of circuits, reflexes, motor control, proprioceptive and nociceptive processes, and referred pain that perpetuates dentomandibular sensorimotor dysfunction.[2] As the muscles work against each other to adapt to occlusal imbalances, trigger points develop. These contribute to referred pain, which is experienced in other areas. It is highly likely that individuals with dentomandibular sensorimotor dysfunction have multiple trigger points in the muscles surrounding the head, neck, and jaw (Figures 2.6

What is a trigger point?

A trigger point is a hyperirritable spot formed only in the muscles that is painful. It is called a trigger point because it "triggers" a painful response. Located in a taut band of muscles fibers, a trigger point is the most tender point in the band. However, more than merely tender nodules, trigger points not only affect the muscle where they are located, but also cause "referred pain" in tissues supplied by nerves.

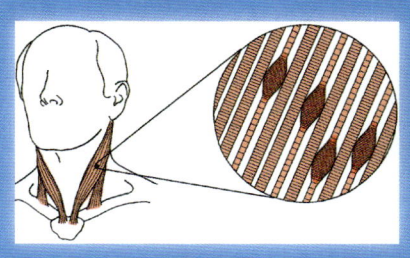

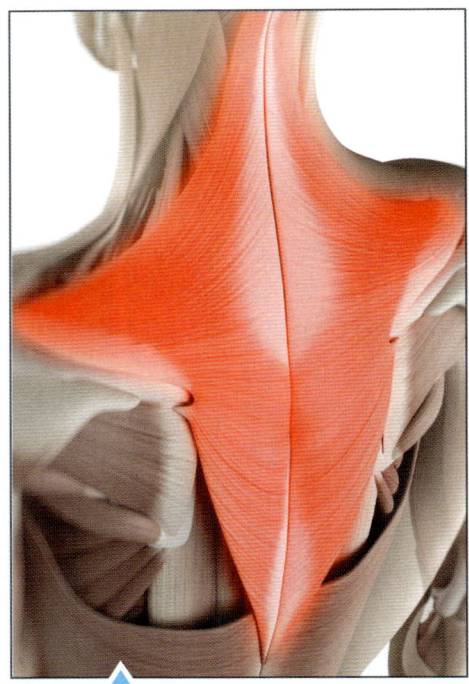

FIGURE 2.6. The trapezius muscle is innervated by the accessory nerve CN XI and the ventral rami of the third (C3) and fourth (C4) cervical nerves. Sensation, including pain and proprioception, travel via the C3 and C4 ventral rami.

constantly receiving nerve signals. As a result, it is not uncommon for patients with TMJ/D to experience severe and chronic pain and disability.[20] Injuries, trauma, or inflammation to the dentomandibular and craniofacial tissues (e.g., muscles) affect the transmission, modulation, and adaptation of nociceptive signals in the brain stem, which underlies pain in the face, mouth, and head.[21] In fact, orofacial and dentomandibular pain often involves inflammation of the soft tissues in this area. Also, peripheral and central neural processes are involved with this pain.[22]

through 2.8).[19] Nociceptive input from peripheral tender muscles can result in central sensitization and chronic headache conditions.

Due to the fact that all of these areas are similarly controlled by the brachial arch cranial nerves that begin in the brain stem, they are

If abnormal, force related conditions that affect the processes of non-neural glial cells in the nervous system are not addressed, peripheral and central sensitization can play a role in an individual's ongoing discomfort.[22] Glial receptors are stimulated during physiological conditions, releasing glutamate and playing an active role in pain perception.[23-26] Glutamate-evoked jaw or neck muscle pain is linked to several clinical conditions in the

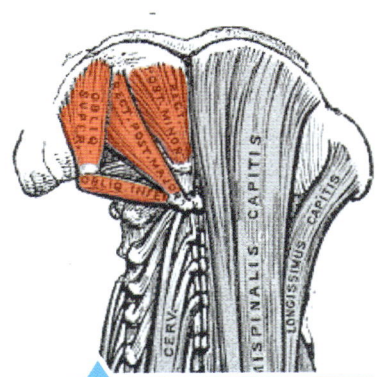

FIGURE 2.7. The suboccipital muscle is palpated by applying five pounds of pressure posterior to anterior, and medially.

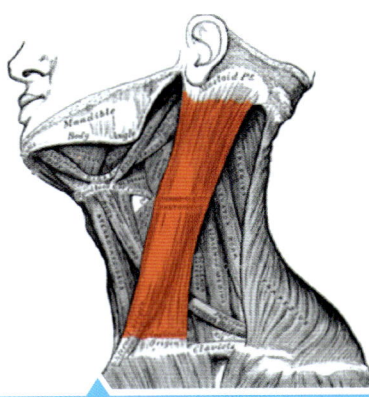

FIGURE 2.8. The sternocleidomastoid muscle acts to flex and rotate the head. When acting alone, it tilts the head to its own side and rotates it to the opposite side. When both act together, they flex the neck, raise the sternum, and assist in forced respiration.

craniofacial and cervical regions.[27] When deep tissue trauma and pain occur, altered muscle activity in the orofacial and cervical regions (e.g., abnormal forces, bruxism, clenching) are likely to be involved in altered neuromuscular activity.

■ Implications for Dentomandibular and Headache Pain Treatments

It has long been understood that headaches are mediated by the trigemino-cervical nucleus. Headache pain results from aggravating stimulation of the nerve endings that unite within this area, or from irritation to the nerves themselves.[28] However, referred pain from disorders occurring elsewhere in the body—such as the dentomandibular region—can be perceived as headache. This is a result of the convergence between trigeminal afferents and those of the cervical nerves in the trigemino-cervical nucleus.[29]

Since only structures that are innervated by certain trigeminal branches are known to cause headache—including the muscles, joints, and ligaments in the mandible and maxilla—the role of dentomandibular sensorimotor dysfunction in headache pain becomes clear.[30] Comorbidities of tension and migraine headaches involve neurologic disorders that cause recurrent or persistent pain.[31] Individuals with TMJ/D and facial pain symptoms have demonstrated significantly greater numbers of headache symptoms than those who do not. Their headaches were also more severe.[32]

Clearly, the essence of force related dental disease, including its effects on the head, orofacial, and dentomandibular areas, is determined by the manner in which abnormal forces are managed, sensed, and adapted to.[1-7] Due to the role neurology plays in the disruptive processes associated with dentomandibular sensorimotor dysfunction, establishing normal function and relieving patients of pain symptoms requires that the neurology, muscle activity, and brain chemistry be "reset."[21,22] Dentists can better manage individuals experiencing debilitating pain by rehabilitating proper biological, physical, and neurophysiological functions.

A crucial aspect of rehabilitation is creating a balanced foundation, which involves more than balancing forces. Rather, it requires adherence to a specific protocol in which the symmetry of the muscles and joints is the initial focal point of care. This pathway to care can then enable dentists to treat dentomandibular sensorimotor dysfunction. It also enables them to relieve patients of its associated symptoms by controlling muscle forces and force balance, and rehabilitating and restoring normal function and range of motion. They can also achieve relief by resetting engram patterns of pain, dysfunction, and muscle activity. Balancing the dental foundation requires balancing the muscles, joints, and teeth, as well as controlling the proprioceptive feedback loops.

In conjunction with this, rehabilitation of musculoskeletal injuries, including those resulting from masticatory forces, is effective when provided in a timely and appropriate manner. Whether in sports or general physical rehabilitation, therapeutic protocol progresses sequentially to control pain, restore range of motion, retrain the neuromuscular complex, and re-establish normal function and activity.[33] The commonly used therapeutic modalities include ultrasound and electrical stimulation.[34] Additionally, research has shown that habit reversal techniques may be promising in reducing dentomandibular-related pain.[4]

■ Embracing New Opportunities for Assessment and Therapy

High-level sports medicine has recognized that rehabilitation programs should be designed to include a proprioceptive component. This component would address cognitive programming and brainstem activity to promote dynamic joint and functional stability. Given what is understood about the trigeminal nerve, as well as the muscles of the dentomandibular complex that it affects and the pain symptoms individuals experience as a result of abnormal forces in this area, dentistry can embrace assessment and therapeutic modalities that complete a crucial task. They encompass afferent feedback to the brain, nerve pathways, and neuromuscular feedback as a means to assess and relieve the causes of an individual's pain and provide a long-term foundation of health and well-being.[35]

For example, professional athletes benefit from specialized doctors, therapists, and trainers. They incorporate a protocol of diagnostics, treatment, and rehabilitation procedures, with a plan to enhance their skills as professional healers. Following initial recovery, athletes undergo specific work and/or therapy that enable them to regain the fitness or health required for normal function.[36]

Just as an orthopedist must balance the rehabilitation of a patient's muscles, ligaments, and joints with the development of a planned prosthesis, dentists can approach rehabilitation beginning with the most adaptable tissues: the muscles. They then proceed to joint rehabilitation, and they finalize therapy with dental treatment of the teeth. Although many problems with the dental foundation have a chicken or the egg etiology, all therapy for dental foundation or bite imbalance can be approached comprehensively, dealing with all foundational elements in order to achieve success.

When all the elements of teeth, muscles, joints, neurology, pain, and force balance are addressed, the patient will have the best chance for an excellent outcome. Similar to the proven modalities and methods of sports medicine, this process can begin with imaging and assessment technologies, along with updated treatment paradigms.[37] Sports rehabilitation methods begin with basic measures and progress through rehabilitation with quantitative feedback to evaluate physiologic response to therapy.[38] By following a similar functional progression, dentists can ensure patients are appropriately responding to treatment and managing their condition.

This rehabilitation approach is the cornerstone of a medical-dental synergy. It is an innovative assessment and treatment technology now available for dental practices called TruDenta. It enables an objective assessment of muscle and force dysfunction, as well as pain management through physical rehabilitation of the musculoskeletal physiology. The TruDenta system is a unique and complete combination of equipment, technology, software, and therapeutic protocols, all of which have been well developed and tested to help achieve predictable results through straightforward, conservative care.

References

1. Junge D. *Oral Sensorimotor Function*. Medico Dental Media International, Inc.: 1998.

2. Sessle BJ. Mechanisms of oral somatosensory and motor functions and their clinical correlates. *J Oral Rehabilitation*. 2006; 33:243-261.

3. Montgomery MW, Shuman L, Morgan A. T-scan dental force analysis for routine dental examination. *Dent Today*. 2011 Jul;30(7):112-4, 116.

4. Glaros AG. Temporomandibular disorders and facial pain: a psychophysiological perspective. *Appl Psycholphysiol Biofeedback*. 2008 Sep;33(3):161-171.

5. Koolstra JH. Dynamics of the human masticatory system. *Crit Rev Oral Biol Med*. 2002;13(4):366-76.

6. Dawson P. *Functional Occlusion: From TMJ to Smile Design*. Canada: Mosby, Inc.; 2007.

7. Hess LA. The relevance of occlusion in the golden age of dentistry. *Inside Dent*.2008; 36-44.

8. Williamson EH, Lundquist W. Anterior guidance: Its effect on electromyographic activity of the temporal and masseter muscles. *J Prosthet Dent*. 1983; 49(6):816.

9. Carlsson GE. Some dogmas related to prosthodontics, temporomandibular disorders and occlusion. *Acta Odontol Scand*. 2010 Nov;68(6):313-22.

10. Singh M, Detamore MS. Biomechanical properties of the mandibular condylar cartilage and their relevance to the TMJ disc. *J Biomech*. 2009 Mar 11;42(4):405-17.

11. Schindler HJ, Rues S, Türp JC, Schweizerhof K, Lenz J. Jaw clenching: muscle and joint forces, optimization strategies. *J Dent Res*. 2007 Sep;86(9):843-7.

12. Simon J. Biomechanically-induced dental disease. *Gen Dent*. 2000 Sep-Oct;48(5):598-605.

13. Kampe T. Function and dysfunction of the masticatory system in individuals with intact and restored dentitions. A clinical, psychological and physiological study. *Swed Dent J Suppl*. 1987;42:1-68.

14. Kerstein RB. Reducing chronic masseter and temporalis muscular hyperactivity with computer-guided occlusal adjustments. *Compend Contin Educ Dent*. 2010 Sep;31(7):530-4, 536, 538.

15. Shankland WE 2nd. The trigeminal nerve. Part I: an overview. *Cranio*. 2000 Oct; 18(4):238-48.

16. Shankland WE 2nd. The trigeminal nerve. Part II: the ophthalmic division. *Cranio*. 2001 Jan; 19(1):8-12.

17. Shankland WE 2nd. The trigeminal nerve. Part III: the maxillary division. *Cranio*. 2001 Apr; 19(2):78-83.

18. Shankland WE 2nd. The trigeminal nerve. Part IV: the mandibular division. *Cranio*. 2001 Jul; 19(3):153-61.

19. Fernandez-de-las-Penas C, Cuadrado ML, Arendt-Nielson L, Simons DG, Pareja JA. Myofacial trigger points and sensitization: an updated pain model for tension-type headache. *Cephalalgia*. 2007 May;27(5):383-93. [Epub 2007 May 14]

20. Velly AM, Look JO, Carlson C, Lenton PA, Kang W, Holcroft CA, Fricton JR. The effect of catastrophizing and depression on chronic pain--a prospective cohort study of temporomandibular muscle and joint pain disorders. *Pain*. 2011 Oct;152(10):2377-83.

21. Sessle BJ. Recent insights into brainstem mechanisms underlying craniofacial pain. *J Dent Educ*. 2002 Jan;66(1):108-12.

22. Sessle BJ. Peripheral and central mechanisms of orofacial inflammatory pain. *Int Rev Neurobiol*. 2011;97:179-206.

23. Overstreet LS. Quantal transmission: not just for neurons. *Trends Neurosci*. 2005 Feb;28(2):59-62.

24. Peters A. A fourth type of neuroglial cell in the adult central nervous system. *J Neurocytol*. 2004 May;33(3):345-57.

25. Huang YH, Bergles DE. Glutamate transporters bring competition to the synapse. *Curr Opin Neurobiol.* 2004 Jun;14(3):346-52.

26. Volterra A, Steinhäuser C. Glial modulation of synaptic transmission in the hippocampus. *Glia.* 2004 Aug 15;47(3):249-57.

27. Wang K, Sessle BJ, Svensson P, Arendt-Nielsen L. Glutamate evoked neck and jaw muscle pain facilitate the human jaw stretch reflex. *Clin Neurophysiol.* 2004 Jun;115(6):1288-95.

28. Bogduk N. Anatomy and physiology of headache. *Biomed Pharmacother.* 1995; 49(10):435-45.

29. Bogduk N. The neck and headaches. *Neurol Clin.* 2004 Feb;22(1):151-71,vii.

30. Bogduk N. The anatomical basis for cervicogenic headache. *J Manipulative Physiol Ther.* 1992 Jan;15(1):67-70.

31. Robbins MS, Lipton RB. The epidemiology of primary headache disorders. *Semin Neurol.* 2010 Apr;30(2):107-19.

32. Pettingill C. A comparison of headache symptoms between two groups: a TMD group and a general dental practice group. *Cranio.* 1999 Jan;17(1):64-9.

33. Mahan PE, Wilkinson TM, Gibbs CH, et al. Superior and inferior bellies of the lateral pterygoid muscle EMG activity at basic jaw positions. *J Prosthet Dent.* 1983; 50(5):710-718.

34. Chapman BL, Liebert RB, Lininger MR, Groth JJ. An introduction to physical therapy modalities. *Adolesc Med State Art Rev*. 2007 May;18(1):11-23, vii-viii.

35. Lephart SM, Pincivero DM, Giraldo JL, Fu FH. The role of proprioception in the management and rehabilitation of athletic injuries. *Am J Sports Med*. 1997 Jan-Feb;25(1):130-7.

36. Williams RJ 3rd. Getting injured players back on the field. *The New York Times*. January 22, 2011. http://goal.blogs.nytimes.com/2011/01/22/getting-injured-players-back-on-the-field/

37. Cates W, Cavanaugh J. Advances in rehabilitation and performance testing. *Clin Sports Med*. 2009 Jan;28(1):63-76.

38. Borg-Stein J, Zaremski JL, Hanford MA. New concepts in the assessment and treatment of regional musculoskeletal pain and sports injury. *PM R*. 2009 Aug;1(8):744-54.

Chapter 2 Self-Assessment Quiz

1. Clinically managing the conditions and symptoms of dentomandibular sensorimotor dysfunction is dependent upon which of the following?

    a. Controlling pain and inflammation.

    b. Rehabilitating the system to normal function and range of motion.

    c. Dental stabilization of the stomatognathic system.

    d. All of the above.

2. The forces between the teeth via the musculature may be altered when neurology is abnormal.

    a. True.

    b. False.

(cont.)

Chapter 2 Self-Assessment Quiz (cont.)

3. Treating dentomandibular sensorimotor dysfunction can achieve which of the following?

    a. Pain relief.

    b. Restoration of normal function and range of motion.

    c. Both a and b.

    d. None of the above.

4. Which of the following does not describe the mandibular or third division of the trigeminal nerve?

    a. A mixed nerve that conveys afferent fibers and efferent fibers to the masticatory muscles.

    b. Purely sensory and afferent.

    c. Refers pain to other areas within its branches, as well as to other trigeminal divisions.

    d. None of the above.

(cont.)

Chapter 2 Self-Assessment Quiz (cont.)

5. Dentomandibular sensorimotor dysfunction is perpetuated by which of the following?

    a. Proprioceptive and nociceptive processes.

    b. Referred pain.

    c. Dental stabilization.

    d. Both a and b.

3 | The TruDenta System for Assessing and Treating Dentomandibular Sensorimotor Dysfunction

The treatments available for addressing temporomandibular joint disorders (TMJ/D), pain, and dysfunction have evolved over the years. The diagnostics, accuracy of clinical findings, and new therapeutic regimens are also enabling dentists to relieve patients of pain.[1] There has been a recent increase in the understanding of the mechanisms that exacerbate and/or cause pain in the face, head, oral environment, and the joints and muscles in these areas. As a result, dentistry is poised to embrace a new paradigm in the assessment, rehabilitation,

LEARNING OBJECTIVES

After reading this chapter, the reader should be able to:

1. List the therapeutic outcomes expected from using certain treatment modalities for dentomandibular sensorimotor dysfunction.

2. Explain physical and digital/objective steps that can help determine a patient's level of dentomandibular sensorimotor disability.

3. Describe the rationale for assessing and treating dental force imbalances.

and treatment of destructive force related dental problems.

These "foundation" problems must be addressed and controlled at the heart of the problem. This involves the afferent signals from the teeth to the trigeminal cervical nucleus. The trigeminal cervical nucleus is the brainstem pathway in the dentomandibular area that conducts all of the information regarding headache, head and face pain, and TMJ/D-related pain to the patient's thalamus and on to the cortex.[2,3] Therefore, it stands to reason that patients who present with such problems centered in the teeth, muscles, joints, or trigeminal cervical nucleus can be cared for by knowledgeable dentists and realize the greatest opportunity for pain resolution.[2-5]

Fortunately, dentists now can objectively assess the forces causing these problems and systematically treat and monitor their patients who experience symptoms of muscle and force dysfunction. Research and technology developed for, and proven effective in, disciplines like sports medicine and rehabilitation are enabling dentists to address the patient population experiencing the debilitating symptoms of dentomandibular sensorimotor dysfunction. In combination with neuroscience and systematic and objective assessment/monitoring, the TruDenta system allows a comprehensive approach to be applied to treatment.[6-11]

The premise of the TruDenta system is to enable dentists to simply redirect the focus of the examination processes and initial care sequences. In doing this, they can address the underlying parafunctional physiology.[12-19] The evolutionary and revolutionary system is built upon various common concepts. It is based on the concepts of occlusion,[20-23] dental anatomy,[20] mastication physiology,[15,20] oral sensorimotor function,[3,24] and the musculoskeletal anatomy and function of the head and neck.[20,24,25] The care program also has elements of the applied neurology of the afferent and efferent pathways, which are involved with sensation, proprioception, pain, reflex motor control, and compensatory adaptations and engrams of function and parafunction.[26-29]

By utilizing the TruDenta system, dentists can offer their patients the opportunity to deal with their symptoms and problems in a way that assures them of a pathway to long-term predictable health and dental stability. In addition, by addressing the problems at the level of mechanical causation (i.e., dental force related conditions), dentists can expand their care to include excellent results for many individuals with intractable, late, or end stage disorders. These may include severe dental disease, as well as head and neck pain, range of motion disabilities, and accelerated aging. All of this could be related to dysfunction and poorly healed injuries.[30,31]

Fundamentally, once TruDenta treatments have achieved functional and dynamic optimization, then the mechanical aspects of occlusion can be addressed. This rationale stems from the understanding that, generally speaking, any time there is a need to address a patient's symptoms connected to the dental foundation, it is in the individual's best interest to have the foundation stabilized and balanced. This should occur prior to, or as a part of, any treatment for the problem. If any restorative treatment is needed for the patient, the best possible outcome will reside in the approach that builds a balanced foundation as the first step to care.[3,15,23,25]

■ *The Scientifically Proven Components*

The TruDenta® assessment and treatment system is a complete, state-of-the-art system for the assessment, treatment, and management of functional, dynamic force imbalances (Figure 3.1). These imbalances are assessed using a

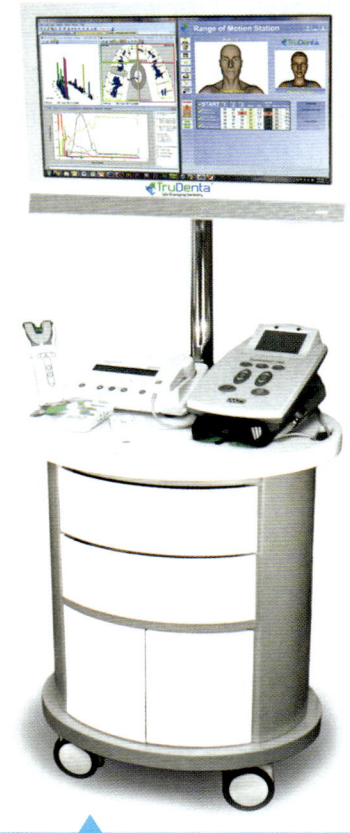

FIGURE 3.1. The TruDenta system is a complete, state-of-the-art system for assessing, treating, and managing functional, dynamic force imbalances.

combination of hardware and software that are supplemented by extensive clinical training and ongoing practice implementation assistance. The equipment in the TruDenta system are all devices cleared by the Food and Drug Administration, and they have been utilized in sports medicine rehabilitation for over a decade. Physicians and dentists in hospitals and clinics around the globe utilize this equipment in the routine delivery of care.[32-34]

■ *Examinations and Histories*

As with any diagnostic and clinical treatment protocol, the first step in the TruDenta approach to patient care is the examination. During the examination, the condition(s) that may be amenable to treatment are assessed. The TruDenta system includes a well-described and documented screening and examination protocol that helps to identify those patients who will be responsive to TruDenta treatment and those who will not.[35,36]

The examination process includes a head health, medical, and headache history, as well as a pharmacological assessment. These findings are combined with a standard of care panoramic radiographic examination.[37] Thorough dental, periodontal, airway, orthodontic, and occlusal examinations are also recommended and encouraged.

The panoramic radiograph is utilized to screen for many dental conditions that patients may have, but for the TruDenta assessment and rehabilitation approach, it provides insight into certain areas implicated in dentomandibular dysfunctions and imbalances (Figure 3.2). By reviewing the panoramic radiograph, dentists can confirm their findings. They can also determine the extent of the problems and direct treatment or further testing. Additionally, computed tomography (CT) scans also may be utilized.

For example, screening may suggest the presence of abnormally shaped or sized mandibular condyles. This condition may be due to injury or disease (e.g., degenerative condyles).[38] Some of the most common causes for this degeneration include TMJ capsule, arthritis (i.e., osteoarthritis and rheumatoid arthritis), and avascular necrosis related to injury during growth. Other causes include chronic injury, microtrauma, or rapid deceleration injury (e.g., whiplash), as well as hyperactivity of the muscles of mastication. Additionally, panoramic radiographs and CT scans may identify antegonial notching of the lower border of the mandible, which is related to excessive activity in both frequency and force of the masseters and medial pterygoid muscles.[39] This is often suggestive of a sensorimotor dysfunction, which is related to the parafunctional activity of clenching and/or grinding.

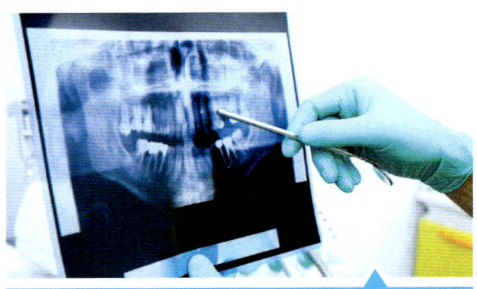

FIGURE 3.2. A panoramic radiograph is utilized to provide insight into certain areas implicated in dentomandibular dysfunctions and imbalances.

Similarly, mandibular asymmetries almost always will establish an asymmetrical mandibular movement related to unbalanced mandibular musculature. This occurs in both anatomically and in compensatory movements. These imbalances and subsequent abnormal development of the mandible can result from asymmetrical muscle function or injury, poor tongue position, airway disorders, and/or dysphagia. They can also result from loss of condylar height from injury of degenerative disease, and/or excessive condylar size related to neoplasm/growth disorder/tumor.[40]

Many of the root causes of dentomandibular sensorimotor dysfunction also contribute to sleep disordered breathing. The TruDenta assessment evaluation seeks to determine if patients suffer from upper airway restrictions caused by excessively large turbinates, nasal polyps, inflammation of the turbinates (e.g., allergic reactions or infection), deviated nasal septum, or other developmental constrictions. All of these constrictions can be related to narrow, V-shaped, underdeveloped, asymmetrical, and/or highly vaulted palates. Airway issues related to dentomandibular sensorimotor dysfunction can result in poor airflow or nasal breathing with resultant decrease or no production during sleep, poor sleep patterns, poor tongue function, and dysphagia. They can also be accompanied by snoring, sleep disturbances, obstructive sleep apnea, as well as poor vascular tone from endothelial dysfunction that results in metabolic disorders, mouth breathing, and its resulting sequelae (e.g., dry mouth, increased acidity, increased periodontal infection, poor oral mucosa and immune management).[41,42]

The examination process also includes muscle palpation (Figures 3.3 and 3.4). This involves locating trigger points. Trigger points can be latent or active, with the latter causing pain and restricting motion.

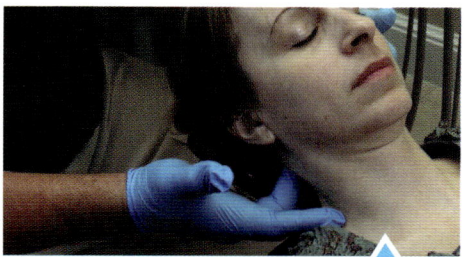

FIGURE 3.3. Manual palpation is used to locate and identify trigger points. Usually there is a taut band in muscles containing trigger points, and a hard nodule can be felt.

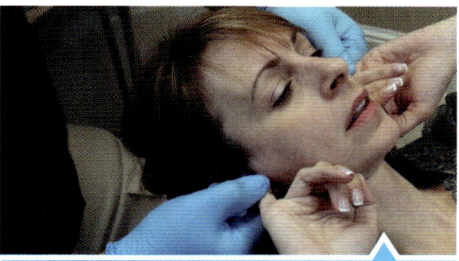

FIGURE 3.4. Pressing on an affected muscle during manual palpation can often refer pain. Clusters of trigger points are not uncommon in some of the larger muscles.

Pain may be merely annoying, or it may be severe, excruciating, debilitating, or even paralyzing. A latent trigger point restricts range of motion, and it is usually experienced as stiffness. Latent trigger points are painful when directly pressed.[43]

Patients may be able to indicate the location of some active trigger points in their head, neck, and shoulders. However, it is the latent trigger points that are most often missed without a thorough muscle palpation examination, since direct pressure is required. The TruDenta system pairs the physical muscle palpation examination with the digital range of motion evaluation. This is because restricted motion indicates the presence of trigger points that require rehabilitation.

■ *The Digital Assessment Modalities*

The physical examination is supplemented by the objective findings from the mandibular range of motion (ROM) disability, cervical range of motion disability (digitally), and a digital force analysis (TruDentaScan). It is important to note that the ROM portion of the assessment process provides objective data that speaks to the American Medical Association guidelines for the rating of pain and disability. These TruDenta assessment devices objectively measure and visually illustrate the cause of patient symptoms as they relate to dentomandibular sensorimotor dysfunctions. Such visualization enhances patient acceptance of treatment and contributes to greater assessment objectivity and treatment monitoring. The TruDenta examination of forces placed on the masticatory system plays a large role in determining the extent of the sensorimotor dysfunction. Abnormal, excessive, or imbalanced forces are reliable indicators of dysfunction and injury.

● *Force Measurement*

In particular, the system uses TruDentaScan digital force measurement (T-Scan) technology to evaluate the amount and imbalance of forces during closure, at closure, and while chewing (Figures 3.5 and 3.6). The T-Scan uses technology that confirms the balance or imbalance of a patient's dental foundation. The use of these force analysis devices incorporates time resolution and plots of the distribution of forces within the occlusion. They have also been shown to be superior to other methods for more accurately measuring occlusal forces.[44-46]

The T-Scan facilitates patient education and screening during evaluation. Its technology also allows dentists to balance the dental foundation as patients proceed along the path of rehabilitation of the muscles and joints. The muscles must be re-

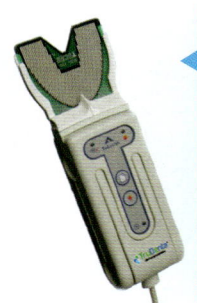

FIGURE 3.5. The TruDentaScan provides a digital force analysis to objectively measure the amount and imbalance of forces during closure, at closure, and while chewing.

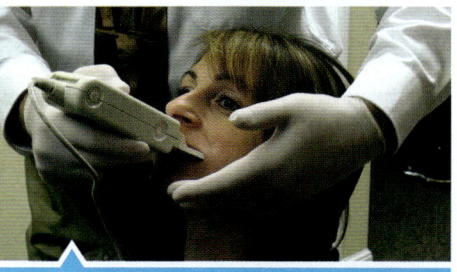

FIGURE 3.6. The TruDentaScan examination of forces placed on the masticatory system plays a large role in determining the extent of dentomandibular sensorimotor dysfunction.

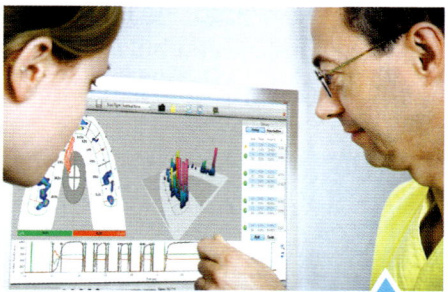

FIGURE 3.7. Objective data obtained from the TruDentaScan facilitates patient education and screening during the evaluation process. It also helps when monitoring patient progress through treatment.

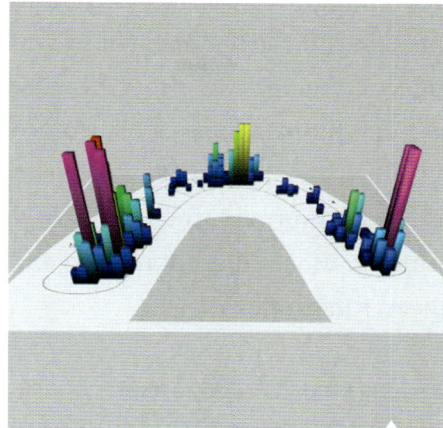

FIGURE 3.9. The 3-dimensional force analysis window displays the forces along the arch in which higher occlusal contact forces are shown as relative peaks of force. Differences in occlusal force can be distinguished by the colors ranging from red (greatest) to blue (lowest), as well as by the height of each column.

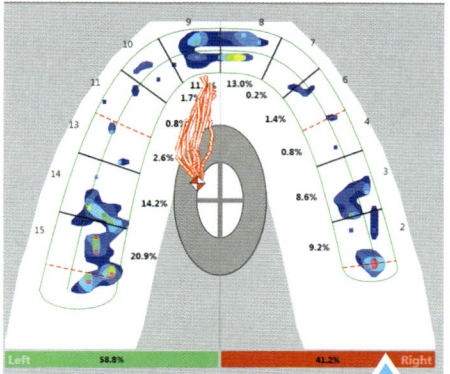

FIGURE 3.8. The 2-dimensional force analysis window displays the forces along the arch, the center of force, the center of force trajectory, and the left/right force balance. This allows dentists to show patients which teeth are generating the most force.

habilitated prior to, or without, the rehabilitation of the joints and joint ligaments. It is only after this has been achieved that further analysis and adjustments can be made to the dentition to harmonize them for normal function.

For example, as patients undergo rehabilitation and the musculoskeletal system improves, dentists use the TruDenta T-Scan technology to monitor progress (Figures 3.7 through 3.9). Subsequently, as needed, they make small but significant changes to the teeth. Initially, these modifications will slightly allow for changes in proprioceptive afferent input to the sensorimotor system. Then, as the somatosensory function improves, the teeth can be brought more and more into balanced function.

- ### Range of Motion Assessment

Another assessment component of the system is the computerized TruDentaROM (Range of Motion) assessment tool (Figure 3.10), which mea-

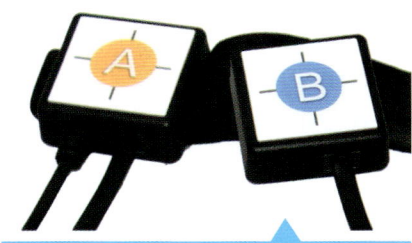

FIGURE 3.10. Using the TruDentaROM, a computerized measuring device, dentists can objectively show the patient their cervical range of motion as expressed in their head movements.

sures the cervical range of motion as expressed in the patient's head movements (Figure 3.11). A cervical range of motion disability can be directly correlated with a mandibular range of motion disability, an imbalance in the

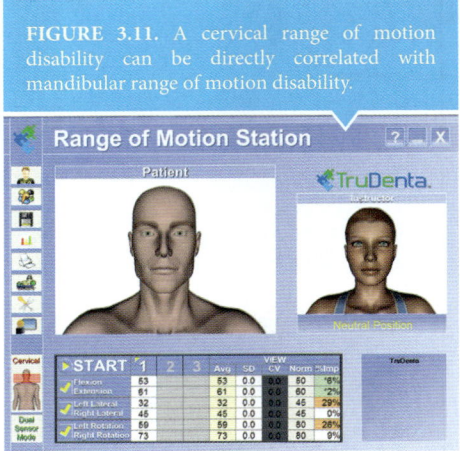

FIGURE 3.11. A cervical range of motion disability can be directly correlated with mandibular range of motion disability.

dental foundation, dysfunction of the jaw, and abnormal neurophysiology of the trigeminal-cervical sensorimotor reflex system. This directly affects the proprioceptive feedback system of the dental occlusion, TMJ, and the muscles of mastication. Measurements made with ROM devices have been shown to be reliable in all movement directions (Figures 3.12 through 3.15), including individuals with soft tissue trauma from whiplash.[47-49]

Limited range of motion equates to dis-

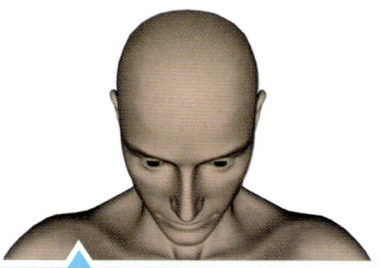

FIGURE 3.12. With a forward flexion of 50°, patients can bring their chin to their chest.

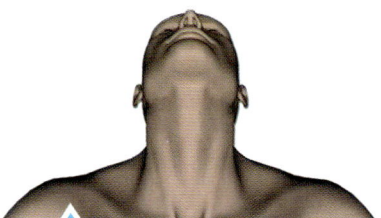

FIGURE 3.13. With an extension of 60°, patients look up and their eyes should be perpendicular to the ceiling.

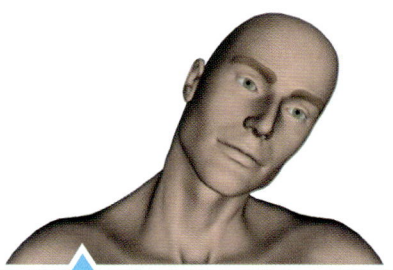

FIGURE 3.14. With a left and right lateral flexion of 45°, patients can bring their ear halfway to the shoulder.

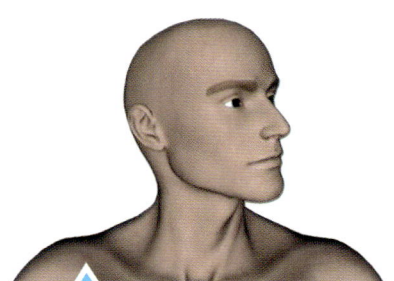

FIGURE 3.15. With a left and right rotation of 80°, patients can bring their chin to their shoulder.

ability. The dentist's ability to objectively measure the range of motion of the head atop the cervical spine greatly enhances patient understanding of their disability. The range of motion examination demonstrates to patients what is normal and where their own mouth, head, and neck are at the time of examination.

A normal opening for an adult is 53 mm to 57 mm. Limited or restricted range of motion (less than 40 mm) is a reduction in an individual's ability for normal range of movement.[50-52] Along with opening movement, an individual should be able to slide their jaw to the left and to the right at least

25 percent of their total mouth opening in a symmetrical fashion.[53]

When restricted movement exists, an imbalance in the system is present, and breakdown of that system is likely to occur. In the case of the mouth range of opening, when an individual cannot open their mouth very far, the muscles supporting the TMJ are restricted due to pain, strain, inflammation, swelling, injury, disease, or another cause.[54,55]

The range of motion measurement also includes a review of the joint noises and vibrations. This is because any noise in the TMJs is intimately related to restriction in the mandibular range of motion. Normal TMJs do not make sounds or have vibrations. If the joints are not smooth and/or quiet, this indicates dysfunction.[56]

■ The Rehabilitation Modalities

Once the condition is determined to be amenable to TruDenta therapy protocols, patients receive a series of treatment therapies. These include using a proprietary combination of frequency, time, and modulation of low level laser therapy, therapeutic ultrasound, and microcurrents to control muscle forces and force balance, rehabilitate and restore normal function and range of motion, and reset engram patterns of pain, dysfunction, and muscle activity. Balancing the muscles, joints, and teeth, as well as controlling the proprioceptive feedback loops, achieves normal function and a stable foundation.

The TruDenta treatment modalities are well described in textbooks and literature that specifically teach many of the principles that underpin the foundation of the TruDenta protocol. Clinical trial outcomes, which were performed during the FDA clearance process of the therapeutic modalities used in the TruDenta treatment plan, support its efficacy.

The multiple TruDenta treatment modalities are a proven combination of sports medicine rehabilitation and advanced dentistry techniques. This combination has been shown to speed the healing of joints and force related traumas.[6-11] The TMJ responds to therapies in a similar manner as ankles, knees, shoulders, and other joints, which are typically treated in sports medicine.

● Therapeutic Ultrasound

The goal of therapeutic ultrasound treatment is to return circulation to sore, strained muscles through increased blood flow and heat (Figure 3.16). Another goal is to break up scar tissue and deep adhesions through sound waves.[9,57]

Therapeutic exposure to ultrasound reduces trigger point sensitivity and has been indicated as a useful clinical tool for managing myofacial pain.[9] Additionally, ultrasound also has been shown to evoke antinociceptive effects on trigger points.[57]

● Transcutaneous Electrical Stimulation

Sub-threshold microcurrent stimulation reduces muscle spasm and referral

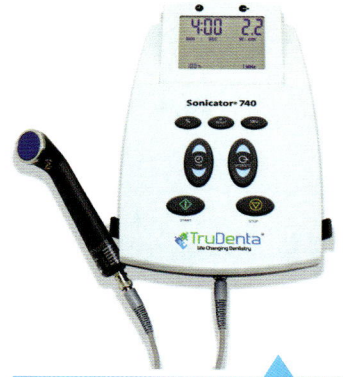

FIGURE 3.16. Therapeutic ultrasound returns circulation to sore, strained muscles and helps to break up scar tissue and deep adhesions.

pain through low electrical signal (Figures 3.17 and 3.18). It also decreases lactic acid build-up and encourages healthy nerve stimulation.[11,58] In particular, microcurrent electrotherapy has been shown to help increase mouth opening significantly.[58]

● Low Level Laser/Light Therapy

Low level laser/light therapy decreases pain and inflammation, accelerates healing of muscle and joint tissue 25 to 35 percent faster than usual, and reconnects neurological pathways of nerves to the brain stem, thereby

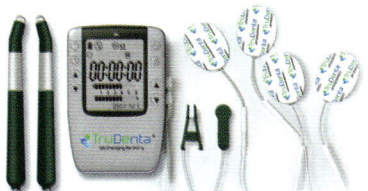

FIGURE 3.17. Sub-threshold microcurrent stimulation reduces muscle spasm and referral pain.

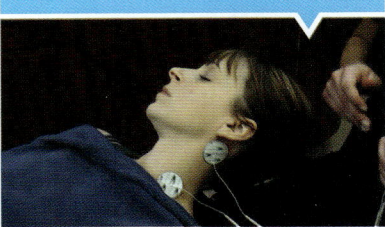

FIGURE 3.18. Sub-threshold microcurrent stimulation helps to increase mouth opening significantly.

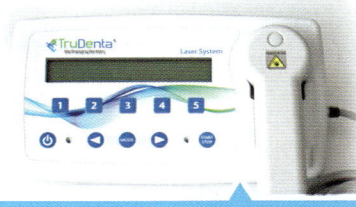

FIGURE 3.19. Low level laser therapy decreases pain and inflammation and accelerates muscle and joint healing.

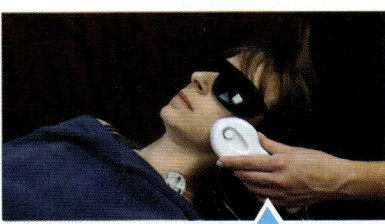

FIGURE 3.20. Low level laser therapy, in combination with electrical stimulation, helps improve mouth opening in patients with TMJ/D.

inhibiting pain (Figures 3.19 and 3.20).[7,8,59-61]

Low level laser therapy, in combination with electrical stimulation, has been shown to improve mouth opening in patients diagnosed with TMJ/D.[56] It decreases pain by promoting the musculoskeletal system's natural healing ability. It also promotes stability of the TMJ.[7,8]

● *Manual Muscle/Trigger Point Therapy*

Manual trigger point therapy decreases and eliminates pain and tension in trigger points (Figure 3.21). This occurs as a result of breaking up muscle knots and increasing blood flow in order to decrease inflammation and pain.[10]

The impetus to treat more than joint/jaw position and dental conditions in isolation comes from the need for predictability and conservative care. Additionally, direct care of the musculature, in conjunction with known systems of jaw position and dental occlusion, can reduce pain, speed recovery times, increase stability, and

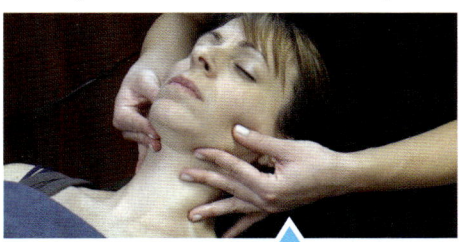

FIGURE 3.21. Manual trigger point therapy decreases and eliminates pain and tension in trigger points.

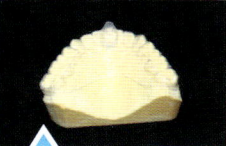

FIGURE 3.22. The purpose of the rehabilitation orthotic is to allow symmetry for joint and muscle rehabilitation, as well as reduce muscle activity of closure muscles.

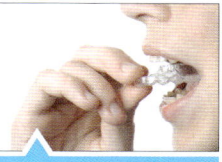

FIGURE 3.23. The goal is for patients to wear the orthotic every night or during normal sleep for between 6 and 12 months, depending on the patient's condition.

reduce the need for pharmaceuticals and radical dental procedures.

Therefore, the TruDenta rehabilitation approach also includes a dentist monitored homecare kit/deprogrammer and intraoral orthotic (Figures 3.22 and 3.23). Overall, the TruDenta assessment and rehabilitation approach addresses dental foundation problems, as well as those associated with dentomandibular sensorimotor dysfunction, through the development of an appropriate pathway to care.

References

1. Dym H, Israel H. Diagnosis and treatment of temporomandibular disorders. *Dent Clin North Am*. 2012 Jan;56(1):49-61.

2. Bogduk N. The neck and headaches. *Neurol Clin*. 2004 Feb;22(1):151-71, vii.

3. Sessle BJ. Mechanisms of oral somatosensory and motor functions and their clinical correlates. *J Oral Rehabil*. 2006 Apr. 33(4):243-61.

4. American Dental Association. Dentists: Doctors of Oral Health. http://www.ada.org/4504.aspx. Accessed July 3, 2012.

5. Fricton JR, Okeson JP. Broad support evident for the emerging specialty of orofacial pain. *Tex Dent J*. 2000 Jul; 117(7):22-5.

6. Cameron MH. *Physical Agents in Rehabilitation*, 3rd Edition. Saunders: 2009.

7. Öz S, Gökçen-Röhlig B, Saruhanoglu A, Tuncer EB. Management of myofacial pain: low-level laser therapy versus occlusal splints. *J Craniofac Surg*. 2010 Nov; 21 (6): 1722-8.

8. Marini I, Gatto MR, Bonetti GA. Effects of superpulsed low-level laser therapy on temporomandibular joint pain. *Clin J Pain*. 2010 Sep; 26(7): 611-6.

9. Srbely JZ, Dickey JP. Randomized controlled study of the antinociceptive effect of ultrasound on trigger point sensitivity: novel applications in myofacial therapy? *Clin Rehabil*. 2007 May; 21(5): 411-7.

10. Aguilera FJ, Martin DP, Masanet RA, Botella AC, Soler LB, Morell FB. Immediate effect of ultrasound and ischemic compression techniques for the treatment of trapezius latent myofascial trigger points in healthy subjects: a randomized controlled study. *J Manipulative Physiolo Ther*. 2009 Sep; 32(7): 515-20.

11. Zuim PRJ, Garcia AR, Turcio KHL, Hamata MM. Evaluation of microcurrent electrical nerve stimulation (MENS) effectiveness on muscle pain in temporomandibular disorders patients. *J Appl Oral Sci*. 2006; 14(1): 61-6.

12. Shankland WE 2nd. The trigeminal nerve. Part III: the maxillary division. *Cranio*. 2001 Apr; 19(2):78-83.

13. Shankland WE 2nd. The trigeminal nerve. Part IV: the mandibular division. *Cranio*. 2001 Jul; 19(3):153-61.

14. Simon J. Biomechanically-induced dental disease. *Gen Dent*. 2000 Sep-Oct;48(5):598-605.

15. Kampe T. Function and dysfunction of the masticatory system in individuals with intact and restored dentitions. A clinical, psychological and physiological study. *Swed Dent J Suppl*. 1987;42:1-68.

16. Fernandez-de-las-Penas C, Cuadrado ML, Arendt-Nielson L, Simons DG, Pareja JA. Myofascial trigger points and sensitization: an updated pain model for tension-type headache. *Cephalalgia*. 2007 May;27(5):383-93. Epub 2007 May 14.

17. Peters A. A fourth type of neuroglial cell in the adult central nervous system. *J Neurocytol.* 2004 May;33(3):345-57.

18. Huang YH, Bergles DE. Glutamate transporters bring competition to the synapse. *Curr Opin Neurobiol.* 2004 Jun;14(3):346-52.

19. Volterra A, Steinhäuser C. Glial modulation of synaptic transmission in the hippocampus. *Glia.* 2004 Aug 15;47(3):249-57.

20. Dawson P. *Functional Occlusion: From TMJ to Smile Design.* Canada: Mosby, Inc.; 2007.

21. Hess, LA. The relevance of occlusion in the golden age of esthetics. *Inside Dent.* 2008:38-44.

22. McNeill C. Occlusion: what it is and what it is not. *J Calif Dent Assoc.* 2000 Oct;28(10):748-58.

23. Okeson JP. *Management of Temporomandibular Disorders and Occlusion*, 6th Edition. Mosby: 2008.

24. Junge D. *Oral Sensorimotor Function.* Medico Dental Media International, Inc.: 1998.

25. Koolstra JH. Dynamics of the human masticatory system. *Crit Rev Oral Biol Med.* 2002;13(4):3.

26. Bogduk N. Anatomy and physiology of headache. *Biomed Pharmacother*. 1995; 49(10):435-45.

27. Sessle BJ. Recent insights into brainstem mechanisms underlying craniofacial pain. *J Dent Educ*. 2002 Jan;66(1):108-12.

28. Sessle BJ. Peripheral and central mechanisms of orofacial inflammatory pain. *Int Rev Neurobiol*. 2011;97:179-206.

29. Lerman MD. The muscle engram: the reflex that limits conventional occlusal treatment. *Cranio*. 2011 Oct; 29(4):297-303.

30. Lephart SM, Pincivero DM, Giraldo JL, Fu FH. The role of proprioception in the management and rehabilitation of athletic injuries. *Am J Sports Med*. 1997 Jan-Feb;25(1):130-7.

31. Borg-Stein J, Zaremski JL, Hanford MA. New concepts in the assessment and treatment of regional musculoskeletal pain and sports injury. *PM R*. 2009 Aug;1(8):744-54.

32. Santos JD, de Oliveira SM, da Silva FM, Nobre MR, Osava RH, Riesco ML. Low-level laser therapy for pain relief after episiotomy: a double-blind randomised clinical trial. *J Clin Nurs*. 2012 May 30;10:1365-2702. [Epub ahead of print]

33. Wakefield RJ, D'Agostino MA, Naredo E, et al. After treat-to-target: can a targeted ultrasound initiative improve RA outcomes? *Postgrad Med J*. 2012 Aug;88(1042): 482-6.

34. Lin YC, Lentz FA. Distribution and response evoked by microstimulation of thalamus nuclei in patients with dystonia and tremor. *Chin Med J* (Engl). 1994 Apr; 107(4):265-70.

35. Straub-Morarend CL, Marshall TA, Holmes DC, Finkelstein MW. Informational resources utilized in clinical decision making: common practices in dentistry. *J Dent Educ*. 2011 Apr;75(4):441-52.

36. Huff K, Huff M, Farah C. Ethical decision-making for multiple prescription dentistry. *Gen Dent*. 2008 Sep-Oct;56(6):538-47.

37. Epstein JB, Caldwell J, Black G. The utility of panoramic imaging of the temporomandibular joint in patients with temporomandibular disorders. *Oral Surg Oral Med Oral Pathol Oral Radiol Endod*. 2001 Aug;92(2):236-9.

38. Magnusson C, Nilsson M, Magnusson T. Degenerative changes in human temporomandibular joints in relation to occlusal support. *Acta Odontol Scand*. 2010 Sep;68(5):305-11.

39. Becker MH, Coccaro PJ, Converse JM. Antegonial notching of the mandible: an often overlooked mandibular deformity in congenital and acquired disorders. *Radiology*. 1976 Oct;121(1):149-51.

40. Tripathi T, Srivastava D, Rai P, Singh H. Asymmetric Class III dentofacial deformities-widening the horizon. *Orthodontics* (Chic.). 2012;13(1):e162-80.

41. Simmons JH. Neurology of sleep and sleep-related breathing disorders and their relationships to sleep bruxism. *J Calif Dent Assoc.* 2012 Feb;40(2):159-67.

42. Bektas D, Cankaya M, Livaoglu M. Nasal obstruction may alleviate bruxism related temporomandibular joint disorders. *Med Hypotheses.* 2011 Feb;76(2):204-5. [Epub 2010 Oct 30]

43. Wright EF. Referred craniofacial pain patterns in patients with temporomandibular disorder. *J Am Dent Assoc.* 2000 Sep;131(9):1307-15.

44. Koos B, Godt A, Schille C, Göz G. Precision of an instrumentation-based method of analyzing occlusion and its resulting distribution of forces in the dental arch. *J Orofac Orthop.* 2010 Nov; 71(6):403-10.

45. Garg AK. Analyzing dental occlusion for implants: Tekscan's TScan III. *Dent Implantol Update.* 2007 Sep; 18(9):65-70.

46. Koos B, Holler J, Schille C, Godt A. Time-dependent analysis and representation of force distribution and occlusion contact in the masticatory cycle. *J Orofac Orthop.* 2012 May; 73(3):204-14.

47. Audette I, Dumas JP, Côté JN, DeSerres SJ. Validity and between-day reliability of the cervical range of motion (CROM) device. *J Orthop Sports Phys Ther.* 2010 May;40(5):318-23.

48. Williams MA, McCarthy CJ, Chorti A, Cooke MW, Gates S. A systematic review of reliability and validity studies of methods for measuring active and passive cervical range of motion. *J Manipulative Physiol Ther.* 2010 Feb; 33(2):138-55.

49. Williams MA, Williamson E, Gates S, Cooke MW. Reproducibility of the cervical range of motion (CROM) device for individuals with sub-acute whiplash associated disorders. *Eur Spine J.* 2012 May;21(5):872-8.

50. Placko G, Bellot-Samson V, Brunet S, Guyot L, Richard O, Cheynet F, Chossegros C, Ouaknine M. [Normal mouth opening in the adult French population]. *Rev Stomatol Chir Maxillofac.* 2005 Nov;106(5):267-71.

51. Gallagher C, Gallagher V, Whelton H, Cronin M. The normal range of mouth opening in an Irish population. *J Oral Rehabil.* 2004 Feb;31(2):110-6.

52. Zawawi KH, Al-Badawi EA, Lobo SL, Melis M, Mehta NR. An index for the measurement of normal maximum mouth opening. *J Can Dent Assoc.* 2003 Dec;69(11):737-41.

53. Mapelli A, Galante D, Lovecchio N, Sforza C, Ferrario VF. Translation and rotation movements of the mandible during mouth opening and closing. *Clin Anat.* 2009 Apr;22(3):311-8.

54. Gupta SK, Rana AS, Gupta D, Jain G, Kalra P. Unusual causes of reduced mouth opening and its suitable surgical management: Our experience. *Natl J Maxillofac Surg.* 2010 Jan;1(1):86-90.

55. Reiter S, Winocur E, Gavish A, Eli I. [Severe limitation of mouth opening]. *Refuat Hapeh Vehashinayim.* 2004 Oct;21(4):36-46, 95.

56. Christensen LV. Physics and the sounds produced by the temporomandibular joints. Part I. *J Oral Rehabil.* 1992 Sep;19(5):471-83.

57. Srbely JZ, Dickey JP, Lowerison M, Edwards AM, Nolet PS, Wong LL. Stimulation for myofascial trigger points with ultrasound induces segmental antinociceptive effects: a randomized controlled study. *Pain.* 2008 Oct 15;139(2):260-6. [Epub 2008 May 27]

58. Dijkstra PU, Kalk WW, Roodenburg JL. Trismus in head and neck oncology: a systematic review. *Oral Oncol.* 2004 Oct;40(9):879-89.

59. Fikácková H, Dostálová T, Vosická R, Peterová V, Navrátil L, Lesák J. Arthralgia of the temporomandibular joint and low-level laser therapy. *Photomed Laser Surg.* 2006 Aug;24(4):522-7.

60. Núñez SC, Garcez AS, Suzuki SS, Ribeiro MS. Management of mouth opening in patients with temporomandibular disorders through low-level laser therapy and transcutaneous electrical neural stimulation. *Photomed Laser Surg.* 2006 Feb;24(1):45-9.

61. Chow RT, Johnson MI, Lopes-Martins RA, Bjordal JM. Efficacy of low-level laser therapy in the management of neck pain: a systematic review and meta-analysis of randomized placebo or active-treatment controlled trials. *Lancet.* 2009 Dec 5;374(9705):1897-908. [Epub 2009 Nov 13]

Chapter 3 Self-Assessment Quiz

1. Afferent and efferent pathways are involved with which of the following?

    a. Sensation.

    b. Proprioception.

    c. Engrams of function and parafunction.

    d. All of the above.

2. The TruDenta system was developed based on common concepts in which of the following areas?

    a. Occlusion.

    b. Applied neurology of afferent and efferent pathways.

    c. Both a and b.

    d. None of the above.

(cont.)

Chapter 3 Self-Assessment Quiz (cont.)

3. Muscle palpation involves locating latent and active trigger points that could restrict range of motion.

    a. True.

    b. False.

4. Digital analysis of forces is performed using which of the following TruDenta system components?

    a. Microcurrent.

    b. T-Scan.

    c. Ultrasound.

    d. Low level laser.

(cont.)

Chapter 3 Self-Assessment Quiz (cont.)

5. Which of the following is not true about the TruDenta treatment modalities?

    a. They have been shown to speed the healing of joints and force related traumas.

    b. They include a proprietary combination of low level laser therapy, therapeutic ultrasound, and microcurrents.

    c. They are devices cleared by the FDA.

    d. None of the above.

4 Life Changing Dentistry: Implications for the TruDenta Pathway to Care

Currently, dental patients can benefit from an enhanced level of care, greater oral health, and overall well-being. Those experiencing any of the multiple symptoms of dentomandibular sensorimotor dysfunction can also benefit from dentistry's ability to help resolve their painful conditions. Dentists can treat patients presenting with problems based in the teeth, muscles of the neck, head and face, or jaw joints. Therefore, their patients can experience relief and life-changing results.[1,2] The TruDenta system and pathway to care enable the restoration of balance, functional harmony, and stability to a patient's dental foundation in a straight forward manner.

The TruDenta care program can treat many different aspects of dentomandibular sensorimotor dysfunction. The program can also treat the spectrum of disorders

LEARNING OBJECTIVES

After reading this chapter, the reader should be able to:

1. Describe how the TruDenta care program approaches treatment of dentomandibular sensorimotor dysfunction.

2. Discuss the indications for which the TruDenta care program may be appropriate.

3. Review the TruDenta rehabilitation process.

that are generally attributed to the stimulus and response involved in the orofacial, head, and neck areas via applied neurology and musculature. Such treatment is supported by the TruDenta approach of addressing the afferent signals from the teeth to the trigeminal cervical nucleus. It also addresses those from the brainstem pathway, which conducts all of the information regarding headache, head and face pain, and temporomandibular joint disorders (TMJ/D) related pain to the patient's thalamus and on to the cortex. The dentomandibular area surrounding the teeth and jaws is the point at which a substantial amount of the afferent control into this pathway originates.[1,2]

As a result, TruDenta has numerous indications and applications. Dentists can care for individuals ranging from those suffering from headaches and migraines to those with pain and limitations. They can also care for patients ranging from those with clenching, grinding, and limited range of motion problems to individuals showing early signs of tooth wear or evidence of imbalance and who need dental treatment.

Temporomandibular-type pains are most often associated with other common pains and rarely present alone.[3] Severe headaches or migraine are often found as a comorbid condition along with TMJ/D-type neck, back, and joint pains.[4] Additionally, migraine is the most prevalent primary headache in individuals with TMJ/D.[5] Also, TMJ/D symptoms are more common in those with migraine, tension-type headaches, and chronic daily headaches, compared to people without headaches.[6] Dental foundation problems often co-exist with headache pain, whether chronic or episodic. Therefore, dentists have an opportunity to provide treatment to a large number of individuals who may not have experienced long-lasting and effective pain relief because the underlying cause of the problem has not been addressed.

The TMJ/headache pain connection to dentomandibular sensorimotor dysfunction is a logical basis on which dentists can provide treatment. In comparison, there are other less-obvious yet similarly related conditions that are equally demanding of TruDenta treatment. Individuals with hyperextension/hyperflexion injuries of the cervical spine (i.e., whiplash) often experience TMJ/D symptoms, internal derangement, effusion, and inflammation.[7] Individuals who suffer whiplash also experience such symptoms, including jaw and neck pain, masseter trigger points, and opening and closing jaw muscle hyperactivity.[8] Individualized, patient-focused therapies and rehabilitation have been effective for patients with debilitating symptoms from whiplash.[9] This suggests that the TruDenta strategies may be appropriate care for such individuals.

Patients experiencing orofacial and dentomandibular pain as a result of dental treatments can also benefit from TruDenta treatment. Orthodontic patients may complain of TMJ/D pain that requires resolution either during or after treatment.[10] When there is a risk of flare-ups of persistent periapical lesions following endodontic treatment, patients may experience painful exacerbations when eating and tooth brushing.[11] Due to the fact that the areas affecting this patient pool are directly tied to the trigeminal cervical nucleus, TruDenta treatment may be beneficial in helping to relieve their pain.

Additionally, prosthodontic care also may benefit preoperatively and postoperatively from TruDenta treatment. This includes full-mouth reconstruction, cosmetic prosthodontics procedures, dentures, and implant-supported therapy.

■ The TruDenta Rehabilitation Process

The TruDenta treatment programs, procedures, and patient care enable dentists and their teams to bring "in house" the majority of conservative musculoskeletal care. This pathway to care can be equally directed to pain, headache, and migraine, or to the degenerative sensorimotor dysfunction that destroys the dentition. Overall, TruDenta therapies are applied to patients with many types of dentomandibular sensorimotor dysfunction and force imbalances in the dental foundation.

The TruDenta pathway to care incorporates four parts. These include an in-office rehabilitation treatment, a rehabilitation orthotic, home care system for patient use, and dental force management through occlusal adjustment procedures. The use of all or some of these components is determined by the patient's assessment and level of care for which they are treatment planned. Patients can be classified into one of four levels, depending on assessment findings (Table 4.1).

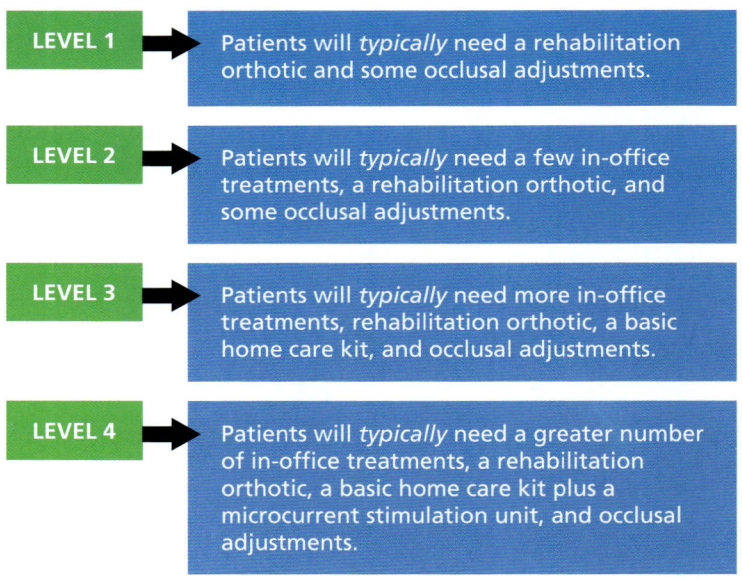

TABLE 4.1. TruDenta Pathway to Care Treatment Levels

LEVEL 1 → Patients will *typically* need a rehabilitation orthotic and some occlusal adjustments.

LEVEL 2 → Patients will *typically* need a few in-office treatments, a rehabilitation orthotic, and some occlusal adjustments.

LEVEL 3 → Patients will *typically* need more in-office treatments, rehabilitation orthotic, a basic home care kit, and occlusal adjustments.

LEVEL 4 → Patients will *typically* need a greater number of in-office treatments, a rehabilitation orthotic, a basic home care kit plus a microcurrent stimulation unit, and occlusal adjustments.

No matter which treatment level patients may be classified as, the goal is to restore balance, functional harmony, and stability to the patient's dental foundation in the most effective and time efficient manner. Balance is restored prior to initiating dental treatment, since periodontal treatments or any other dental procedures on a balanced, stable dental foundation result in longer lasting and more predictable outcomes.[12-14] The need for restorative dentistry is then determined, if appropriate, in a system of balance and stability. This allows the patient to proceed with dental treatment, which will be more predictable and can be accomplished at a comfortable pace, without the urgency of pain.

Every patient is different and requires personalized and individualized treatment, so some patients may respond quickly and others within a few weeks. The patient who presents with an acute problem may proceed quickly through rehabili-

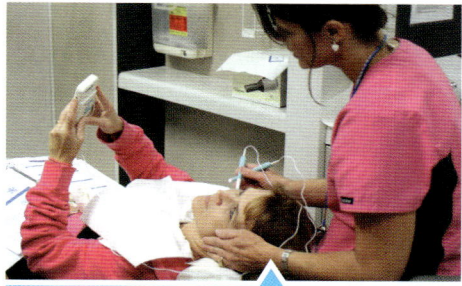

FIGURE 4.1. TruDenta therapy consists of several different and synergistic treatment modalities.

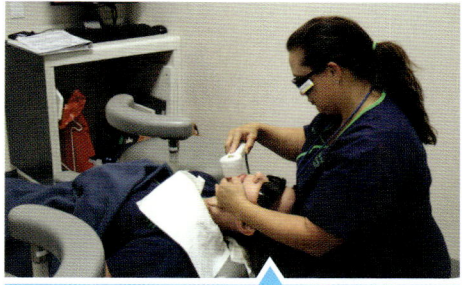

FIGURE 4.2. The TruDenta treatment modalities are usually all utilized in a specific sequence, with specific settings and treatment times.

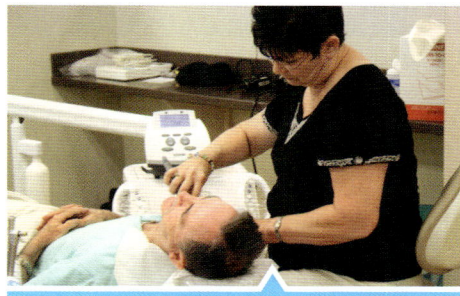

FIGURE 4.3. Typical TruDenta therapy protocol is most appropriate and successful when it progresses sequentially through pain control, restoring range of motion, neuromuscular retraining, and return to normal function.

TABLE 4.2. TruDenta Therapeutic Modalities At-a-Glance

TruDenta Therapeutic Modality	Therapeutic Goal
Ultrasound	Return circulation to sore, strained muscles through increased blood flow and heat, and to break up scar tissue and deep adhesions through sound waves.
Manual Trigger Point Therapy	Decrease and eliminate pain and tension in trigger points; break up muscle knots and increase blood flow; and decrease inflammation and pain.
Alpha-Stim 100	Reduce muscle spasm and referral pain through low electrical signal; decrease lactic acid build-up and encourage healthy nerve stimulation.
Cold Laser Therapy	Decrease pain and inflammation; accelerate healing of muscle and joint tissue; reconnect neurological pathways of nerves to the brain stem, inhibiting pain.

tation to dental restoration. However, patients with limited range of motion in the mandible or cervical spine will require more time to rehabilitate the musculature and reduce pain and disability prior to dental restoration.

TruDenta therapy or treatment appointments are comprised of several different and synergistic treatment modalities (Table 4.2). These include therapeutic ultrasound, transcutaneous electrical stimulation, and low level laser therapy (Figures 4.1 through 4.3). All of these treatments provide predictable results through straightforward, conservative care. The modalities are usually all utilized in a specific sequence, with specific settings and treatment times. Typical therapy protocol is most appropriate and successful when it progresses sequentially through pain control, restoring range of motion, neuromuscular retraining, and return to normal function.[15,16]

As the dentist begins to balance the occlusion, they proceed by balancing the forces applied to the teeth around the dental arch, using both additive and subtractive procedures. This creates and develops a balanced foundation through the rehabilitation process. The TruDenta Scan for analyzing dental force imbalances is used in this process to evaluate numerous characteristics. These include centric occlusion, right and left lateral disclusion, protrusion, hindrances to closure, balance during closure and at full closure, and disclusion locations (e.g., canines, group, posterior, incisors, etc.).

■ *Realizing Life Changing Results*

Patients suffering with obvious pain symptoms appreciate it when dentists and healthcare providers are primarily concerned about enhancing their quality of life. They do this by providing them with an effective way to relieve their pain.[17] This is especially true when practitioners first show them where the pain comes from and then provide the means to experience relief. By treating the pain first through rehabilitation of the dental foundation to a healthy state, restorative dentistry can follow later.

Of course, it is not uncommon for dentists to encounter pain patients reluctant to commit to the recommended level of care. However, presenting an "all or nothing" approach is counterproductive. Dentistry has embraced a phased approach to treatment in order to help patients accept necessary care. In this same manner, dentists can also propose that pain patients begin rehabilitation somewhere.[18]

Although a patient who opts for a lower level of care will most likely achieve a lesser result, doing so does start them in the right direction toward rehabilitation. For example, even just utilizing the orthotic to relieve muscle firing can begin to ease their pain.[19] Additionally, while only one or two therapy appointments may not achieve long-term results, they can be palliative. Care during these appointments can build trust in the process and eventually lead to a commitment to the entire rehabilitation process.[20]

The TruDenta rehabilitation process outlined for each patient level classification provides the most effective and efficient way to restore dental foundation balance and achieve the ideal results. This rehabilitation approach dedicates the appropriate time and frequency of each therapeutic modality to patients, depending on the extent of injury and degree to which their condition has become chronic. These rehabilitation processes have been clinically proven in sports medicine, and additional clinical research will confirm the validity and efficacy of the respective therapeutic protocols.

Based on what is now understood about the mechanisms that exacerbate and/or cause pain in the face, head, oral environment, and the joints and muscles in these areas, dentists can now truly offer life changing treatments. By following the TruDenta pathway to care, dentists and their team members can assess, rehabilitate, and treat destructive force related dental problems. With the Trudenta system, they can also manage the overall health and well-being of their patients.

References

1. Bogduk N. The neck and headaches. *Neurol Clin.* 2004 Feb;22(1):151-71, vii.

2. Sessle BJ. Mechanisms of oral somatosensory and motor functions and their clinical correlates. *J Oral Rehabil.* 2006 Apr. 33(4):243-61.

3. Plesh O, Adams SH, Gansky SA. Temporomandibular joint and muscle disorder-type pain and comorbid pains in a national US sample. *J Orofac Pain.* 2011 Summer;25(3):190-8.

4. Plesh O, Adams SH, Gansky SA. Self-reported comorbid pains in severe headaches or migraines in a US national sample. *Headache.* 2012 Jun;52(6):946-56.

5. Franco AL, Goncalves DA, Castanharo SM, Speciali JG, Bigal ME, Camparis CM. Migraine is the most prevalent primary headache in individuals with temporomandibular disorders. *J Orofac Pain.* 2010 Summer;24(3):287-92.

6. Goncalves DA, Bigal ME, Sales LC, Camparis CM, Speciali JG. Headache and symptoms of temporomandibular disorder: and epidemiological study. *Headache.* 2010 Feb;50(2):231-41. [Epub 2009 Sep. 14]

7. Garcia R Jr, Arrington JA. The relationship between cervical whiplash and temporomandibular joint injuries: an MRI study. *Cranio.* 1996 Jul;14(3):233-9.

8. Friedman MH, Weisberg J. The craniocervical connection: a retrospective analysis of 300 whiplash patients with cervical and temporomandibular disorders. *Cranio*. 2000 Jul;18(3):163-7.

9. DeCarto AA. Rehabilitation approach to treatment of whiplash-associated disorder. *J Amer Chiro Assoc*. 2006 Aug;43(6):6-12.

10. Michelotti A, Iodice G. The role of orthodontics in temporomandibular disorders. *J Oral Rehabil*. 2010 May;37(6):411-29. Epub 2010 Apr 9.

11. Yu VS, Messer HH, Yee R, Shen L. Incidence and impact of painful exacerbations in a cohort with post-treatment persistent endodontic lesions. *J Endod*. 2012 Jan; 38(1):41-6.

12. Dawson P. *Functional Occlusion: From TMJ to Smile Design*. Canada: Mosby, Inc.; 2007.

13. Hess, LA. The relevance of occlusion in the golden age of esthetics. *Inside Dent*. 2008:38-44.

14. McNeill C. Occlusion: what it is and what it is not. *J Calif Dent Assoc*. 2000 Oct;28(10):748-58.

15. Chapman BL, Liebert RB, Lininger MR, Groth JJ. An introduction to physical therapy modalities. *Adolesc Med State Art Rev*. 2007 May;18(1):11-23.

16. Cates W, Cavanaugh J. Advances in rehabilitation and performance testing. *Clin Sports Med*. 2009 Jan;28(1):63-76.

17. Petrie KJ, Frampton T, Large RG, Moss-Morris R, Johnson M, Meechan G. What do patients expect from their first visit to a pain clinic? *Clin J Pain*. 2005 Jul-Aug;21(4):297-301.

18. Eubank JB. Phased treatment for complete dentistry. *Dent Today*. 2008 Jun;27(6):68, 70, 72-3.

19. Attanasio R. Intraoral orthotic therapy. *Dent Clin North Am*. 1997 Apr;41(2):309-24.

20. Levin RP. Developing lifetime relationships with patients: strategies to improve patient care and build your practice. *J Contemp Dent Pract*. 2008 Jan 1;9(1):105-12.

Chapter 4 Self-Assessment Quiz

1. Which of the following are part of the TruDenta approach for treating dentomandibular sensorimotor dysfunction?

    a. Addressing the afferent signals from the teeth to the trigeminal cervical nucleus.

    b. Restoring balance, functional harmony, and stability to a patient's dental foundation.

    c. Both a and b.

    d. None of the above.

2. What type of patient may be amenable to TruDenta treatments?

    a. Individuals experiencing chronic, severe headaches or migraine.

    b. Individuals in need of prosthodontic care.

    c. Individuals with debilitating symptoms from whiplash.

    d. All of the above.

(cont.)

Chapter 4 Self-Assessment Quiz (cont.)

3. According to TruDenta treatment protocol, when is balance restored to the dental foundation?

   a. Prior to initiating restorative dental treatment.

   b. After completing restorative dental procedures.

   c. Whenever necessary.

   d. All of the above.

4. Which of the following is not characteristic of TruDenta therapy?

   a. Therapy is comprised of several different and synergistic treatment modalities.

   b. The same therapeutic modalities are used for all patients, regardless of symptoms.

   c. Therapeutic modalities are used in a specific sequence, with specific settings and treatment times.

   d. None of the above.

(cont.)

Chapter 4 Self-Assessment Quiz (cont.)

5. Which of the following are monitored throughout the TruDenta treatment process?

   a. Pain symptoms.

   b. Trigger point tenderness.

   c. Mandibular range of motion.

   d. All of the above.

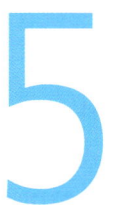

5 | Shifting the Paradigm to Enhance Oral Health and Headache Care Effectiveness

Treatments for temporomandibular joint disorders (TMJ/D), pain, and dysfunction have evolved over the years. Advanced diagnostics, clinical research findings, and new therapeutic regimens have enabled dentists to relieve patients of their painful conditions.[1] As a result, now is the time for dentistry to embrace a new paradigm in the assessment, rehabilitation, and treatment of destructive force related dental problems, including headache pain. The association between oral and systemic diseases has taken center stage in dentistry and medicine. Dentists and their staff are poised to serve as the first line of intervention, or as a collaborate partner, in the assessment and rehabilitation

LEARNING OBJECTIVES

After reading this chapter, the reader should be able to:

1. Describe what patients are looking for when choosing a practice.

2. Summarize characteristics of dentomandibular sensorimotor dysfunction.

3. Discuss the possible impact to a practice of objectively assessing and treating patients with symptoms of dentomandibular sensorimotor dysfunction.

of dentomandibular sensorimotor dysfunction symptoms.[2] Related to the stimulus and response involved in the orofacial area, head, and neck via applied neurology and musculature, dentomandibular sensorimotor dysfunction involves painful conditions, such as headaches, TMJ/D, clenching, and other problems.[3]

Uniting these conditions is the effect of unbalanced or overloaded muscle forces in relation to sensorimotor and somatosensory proprioceptive or nociceptive physiology.[4] Managing these problems depends upon pain and inflammation control, rehabilitation of the system to normal function and range of motion, and orthopedic, orthodontic, and dental stabilization of the stomatognathic system. Similar to the proven modalities and methods used for years in sports medicine, this process can begin with imaging and assessment technologies, as well as updated treatment paradigms.[5] Today's headache and chronic dentomandibular pain sufferers want such an approach.

Research has demonstrated that most patients who are presenting for the first time for treatment of pain expect an explanation of their condition, or to obtain an improved understanding of their pain problem.[6] For such individuals, the most common satisfying outcome is relief or control of pain.

That is essentially the cornerstone of the TruDenta approach to treating and managing dentomandibular sensorimotor dysfunction, along with pain in the greater head, neck, and orofacial area. By first restoring the dynamic soft tissue system and ensuring its proper function, TruDenta creates a pathway for subsequent predictable hard tissue adjustment, if necessary. This is regardless of the occlusal philosophy that a dentist follows, and it is in order to achieve the proper, balanced results and health and well-being.

The TruDenta system enables dentists to objectively assess and predictably treat dental force related conditions. It enables them to actually show patients the potential causes of their symptoms and provide measureable results after a single treatment. The combination of objective assessment and coordinated therapies enables dentists and their team members to provide solutions to patients that measurably improve their lives.

Additionally, the TruDenta methods are unique in their approach to dental force management. Although treating TMJ/D related issues is one aspect of addressing dentomandibular sensorimotor dysfunction, it is not the primary focus of the TruDenta assessment and rehabilitation approach. The first step in dynamic and functional correction is the re-establishment of soft-tissue support and the adaptive mechanism. By doing this, the TruDenta protocol helps to enable dentists to establish the foundation for predictability and stability of subsequent mechanical treatments (ie, restorations). Without a combination approach, the body won't be truly balanced and comfortable through all of the uses of the mouth.

By rehabilitating the musculoskeletal system, the Trudenta system enables an objective assessment of muscle and force dysfunction, as well as pain management. The equipment, technology, software, and therapeutic protocols have been well developed and tested to provide predictable results through straightforward, conservative care. Many of the technologies and treatment modalities used in the TruDenta system were originally developed to treat injuries to the muscles, nerves, ligaments, and tendons of professional athletes. Many of the issues associated with dental force and dentomandibular function are similar. Due to this fact, the expertise of dental practitioners has been combined with sports medicine technology as part of the TruDenta treatment methods.

The success of the TruDenta system rests in the combination of the proven modalities used at specific times, in certain measures, and at certain frequencies. When followed properly in appropriately assessed chronic headache and migraine patients, the protocol has been more than 93 percent successful, according to current users.

Providing patients with comprehensive and modern treatments distinguishes dentists from other practices. It enables the entire dental team to derive personal satisfaction from such life changing dentistry. According to the American Dental Association, dentists' expertise lies not only in treating the teeth and gingival tissues, but also in caring for the muscles of the head, neck, and jaw, as well as the nervous system of the these areas.[7] Assessing and treating patients who suffer from the symptoms of dentomandibular sensorimotor dysfunction further distinguishes dentists from those who merely provide dental restorations. Additionally, the dental profession has reached a time in which an increasing number of educated dental patients choose practices because they are seeking more personalized and attentive care. Incorporating customizable rehabilitative services such as TruDenta that convey respect for the individual's well-being may increase the likelihood that patients will pursue that practice.[8]

The number of patients who make this choice could be significant. It is estimated by those professionals already using the system that the potential patient pool of individuals needing, desiring, and who could benefit from the type of care and rehabilitation provided through the TruDenta system is approximately 50 percent of a practice's existing patients.

The shifting paradigm is gaining momentum. Technological innovations are transforming dentistry and emphasizing its inherently preventative and therapeutic objectives. A few of these innovations include programs, systems, and technologies such as TruDenta, which are designed to establish normal function and relieve painful symptoms. By using such technologies, including the TruDenta system, dentists can provide to their patients a solution and pathway to care that is based on a framework of objective assessment and intervention.

References

1. Dym H, Israel H. Diagnosis and treatment of temporomandibular disorders. *Dent Clin North Am*. 2012 Jan;56(1):49-61.

2. Fricton JR, Okeson JP. Broad support evident for the emerging specialty of orofacial pain. *Tex Dent J*. 2000 Jul; 117(7):22-5.

3. Sessle BJ. Mechanisms of oral somatosensory and motor functions and their clinical correlates. *J Oral Rehabilitation*. 2006; 33:243-261.

4. Glaros AG. Temporomandibular disorders and facial pain: a psychophysiological perspective. *Appl Psycholphysiol Biofeedback*. 2008 Sep;33(3):161-171.

5. Cates W, Cavanaugh J. Advances in rehabilitation and performance testing. *Clin Sports Med*. 2009 Jan;28(1):63-76.

6. Petrie KJ, Frampton T, Large RG, Moss-Morris R, Johnson M, Meechan G. What do patients expect from their first visit to a pain clinic? *Clin J Pain*. 2005 Jul-Aug;21(4):297-301.

7. American Dental Association. Dentists: Doctors of Oral Health. http://www.ada.org/4504.aspx. Accessed July 3, 2012.

8. Levin RP. Developing lifetime relationships with patients: strategies to improve patient care and build your practice. *J Contemp Dent Pract*. 2008 Jan 1;9(1):105-12.

Chapter 5 Self-Assessment Quiz

1. According to this chapter, what are patients seeking when they choose a dental practice?

    a. More personalized and attentive care.

    b. An explanation of their condition.

    c. Relief or control of pain.

    d. All of the above.

2. Which of the following has resulted from advanced diagnostics, clinical research findings, and new therapeutic regimens for dentistry?

    a. Dentists can help to relieve patients of their painful conditions, including headaches.

    b. Dentistry can forgo assessing, rehabilitating, and treating destructive force related dental problems, including headache pain.

    c. Dentists can use a single approach to providing patient care.

    d. Both a and b.

(cont.)

Chapter 5 Self-Assessment Quiz (cont.)

3. What may dentists expect to experience after incorporating a system for objectively assessing and treating dentomandibular sensorimotor dysfunction problems?

    a. A possible increase in the likelihood that patients will pursue that practice.

    b. An estimated 93 percent success rate in assessing and treating patients with chronic headache and migraine pain.

    c. Both a and b.

    d. None of the above.

4. Headaches, TMJ/D, and clenching are united by which of the following?

    a. Unbalanced or overloaded muscle forces.

    b. Somatosensory proprioceptive physiology.

    c. Nociceptive physiology.

    d. All of the above.

(cont.)

Chapter 5 Self-Assessment Quiz (cont.)

5. Which of the following is not a step in the management of dentomandibular sensorimotor dysfunction?

   a. Controlling inflammation.

   b. Rehabilitating the system to normal function and range of motion.

   c. Dental stabilization of the stomatognathic system.

   d. None of the above.

Self-Assessment Quiz Answers

Chapter 1
1: a
2: c
3: d
4: c
5: b

Chapter 2
1: d
2: a
3: c
4: b
5: d

Chapter 3
1: d
2: c
3: a
4: b
5: d

Chapter 4
1: c
2: d
3: a
4: b
5: d

Chapter 5
1: d
2: a
3: c
4: d
5: d

LIST OF TABLES

Chapter 1

Table 1.1   **page 38**
Causes of Dental Disease

Chapter 2

Table 2.1   **page 56**
Conditions and Symptoms Generally
Described as Dentomandibular Sensorimotor
Dysfunction

Table 2.2   **page 58**
Conditions Indicating an Unbalanced System

Table 2.3   **pages 59 through 63**
Components of the Dentomandibular
Sensorimotor Complex

Chapter 4

Table 4.1   **page 114**
TruDenta Pathway to Care Treatment Levels

Table 4.2   **page 116**
TruDenta Therapeutic Modalities At-a-Glance

IMAGE CREDITS

Cover

Cover	Cover	Purchased from INMAGINE®

Chapter 1

Figure 1.1	page 33	Dental Resource Systems, Inc.
Figure 1.2	page 36	A.D.A.M. Images

Chapter 2

Figure 2.1	page 57	Purchased from INMAGINE®
Figure 2.2	page 65	Public domain image
Figure 2.3	page 65	Public domain image
Figure 2.4	page 65	Public domain image
Figure 2.5	page 65	Public domain image
Figure 2.6	page 68	Purchased from INMAGINE®
Figure 2.7	page 69	Public domain image
Figure 2.8	page 69	Public domain image

Chapter 3

Figure 3.1	page 86	Dental Resource Systems, Inc.
Figure 3.2	page 87	Purchased from istockphoto.com
Figure 3.3	page 89	Dental Resource Systems, Inc.
Figure 3.4	page 89	Dental Resource Systems, Inc.
Figure 3.5	page 90	Dental Resource Systems, Inc.
Figure 3.6	page 90	Dental Resource Systems, Inc.
Figure 3.7	page 91	Purchased from istockphoto.com
Figure 3.8	page 91	Dental Resource Systems, Inc.
Figure 3.9	page 91	Dental Resource Systems, Inc.
Figure 3.10	page 92	Dental Resource Systems, Inc.
Figure 3.11	page 92	Dental Resource Systems, Inc.
Figure 3.12	page 93	Dental Resource Systems, Inc.
Figure 3.13	page 93	Dental Resource Systems, Inc.
Figure 3.14	page 93	Dental Resource Systems, Inc.
Figure 3.15	page 93	Dental Resource Systems, Inc.
Figure 3.16	page 95	Dental Resource Systems, Inc.
Figure 3.17	page 96	Dental Resource Systems, Inc.
Figure 3.18	page 96	Dental Resource Systems, Inc.
Figure 3.19	page 96	Dental Resource Systems, Inc.
Figure 3.20	page 96	Dental Resource Systems, Inc.
Figure 3.21	page 97	Dental Resource Systems, Inc.
Figure 3.22	page 97	Dental Resource Systems, Inc.
Figure 3.23	page 97	Purchased from istockphoto.com

Chapter 4

Figure 4.1	page 115	Dental Resource Systems, Inc.
Figure 4.2	page 115	Dental Resource Systems, Inc.
Figure 4.3	page 115	Dental Resource Systems, Inc.

INDEX

A

All-ceramic restorations	34
American Dental Association	40
American Medical Association	89

B

Bruxing/bruxism	32, 34, 39, 69

C

CAD/CAM	31
Caries	30
Cervical range of motion	32, 36, 92
Condylar pathologies	31
Condyles	34, 35, 37, 64, 66, 88
Cone beam computed tomography	31
Cortex	40, 112

D

Dental forces	55
Dentofacial	31
Dentomandibular	32, 37
complex	32
sensorimotor dysfunction	32-34, 42, 55, 56, 64, 67, 70, 84, 87, 88, 97, 111
pain	39, 128
Diagnostics	34
Digital force analysis	89, 90

E

Electrical stimulation/microcurrents	71, 94-96, 116
Endodontics	31, 113

F

Food and Drug Administration	86, 94
Force overload	34

G

Glial cells	68

H

Headache	38, 40, 41, 69, 70, 84, 112, 127
Headache history	86
Head health history	86

I

Inflammation	57, 68, 88, 95, 97, 128
Intervention	30

L

Laser therapy	94, 95, 96, 116, 117
Lateral pterygoid	65, 66

M

Magnetic resonance tomography	34
Mandible	35
Manual muscle therapy	97, 116
Masseter	65, 87
Mastication	40, 64
Masticatory system	34, 90
Malocclusion	34-36
Medical history	86
Microcurrents	94, 95

Migraine	39, 41, 112
Muscle forces	37, 39, 55
Muscle palpation	88, 89

N

National Headache Foundation	41
National Institute of Dental and Craniofacial Research	41
Nerves	
Cranial	64, 68
Cervical	64, 69
Neurophysiology	40, 64, 70
Neuroplasticity	40

O

Occlusion	
adjustments	32, 91, 114
force balanced	37, 129
forces	34, 36, 37, 41, 70, 84, 85
treatments	37, 128
Oral health	29, 30
Orthodontic	57
Orthopedic	57
Orthotic (intraoral)	97, 114

P

Pain	35, 36, 38, 39, 83
chronic	64
head	35, 39, 64, 68, 85
jaw	35, 39, 68, 113
neck	35, 64, 68, 85, 113
orofacial	67, 68, 113
referred	67, 69
symptoms	42
tooth	35, 40
Parafunction	58, 64, 66, 84
Pharmacological assessment	86
Prevention	30
Professional satisfaction	29
Proprioceptive feedback loop	70, 71, 92, 94, 128
Prosthodontics	113

R

Radiographs	30, 87
Range of motion	36, 37, 57, 70, 71, 85, 89, 93, 94, 112, 117, 128
Restorations	32, 36, 58, 66

S

Stomatognathic system	35, 57, 128

T

Technology
- bioluminescence — 30
- diagnostic — 30, 41, 83, 127
- imaging — 30, 31, 128
- innovative — 29
- laser fluorescence — 30
- salivary — 30, 31
- trans-illumination — 30

T-Scan — 32, 90
Temporalis — 65
Temporomandibular joint — 35, 41, 55, 65, 95
    disorder — 39, 41, 70, 83, 96, 112, 127
Thalamus — 40, 112
Tooth decay — 32
Trigeminal cervical nucleus — 32, 35, 40, 55, 64, 69, 84, 112
    Trigeminal nerve — 39, 40, 41, 66, 67, 71
Trigger point — 36, 67, 88, 89, 95, 97, 113, 116

U

Ultrasound — 71, 94, 95, 116, 117

V

Visualization — 90

W

Wear	32, 58, 66
Whiplash	92, 113